No Secrets in a Small Town

Inside the Mind of a Rural Doctor

AJ Yusuf, MD

ISBN (Paperback): 979-8-9957804-0-3

To my parents,

for their love, their sacrifice, and their unwavering belief.

And to Dr. Ward Chambers,

whose life in cardiology set the standard for excellence.

"The Man Himself" is dedicated to Dr. Chambers.

Prologue

There is a side of medicine the public never sees.

It lives in the quiet hum of fluorescent lights at 2:17 a.m., in hallway conversations that never make it into the chart, in decisions made in seconds that echo for years. It lingers in the silence of a physician driving home after losing a patient, replaying every choice, every hesitation, every possibility.

When you walk into a hospital or clinic, you see a receptionist, a nurse, a doctor. You see exam rooms, monitors, a waiting area. You see a visit.

What you don't see is the choreography.

The lab technician running urgent samples while the phone keeps ringing. The ER nurse triaging five crises at once while steadying a frightened family with a calm voice. The hospitalist reviewing charts before sunrise. The administrator calculating how to keep the doors open in a town where the hospital is not just a building. It is survival.

You don't see the ethical debates unfolding in real time.

You don't see the quiet tension between insurance policy and bedside judgment.

You don't see the emotional residue that follows a physician from one room to the next.

I have seen it.

I have learned it.

I have lived it.

This book is an invitation to step behind the curtain and witness the living organism that is modern healthcare. It is beautiful, flawed, heroic, bureaucratic, inspiring, and at times heartbreaking. It runs not on machines or policies, but on people.

If you are not in medicine, this may change the way you experience your next appointment. The next time you sit on an exam table, you may notice more than the white coat. You may sense the invisible machinery and the fragile humanity behind it.

If you work in healthcare, much of this will feel familiar, almost uncomfortably so. You may recognize the exhaustion beneath professionalism, the moral injury that rarely has a name, the quiet triumph of saving a life no one will remember next week. You may disagree at times. Your experience is your own. But I suspect much of this journey will feel shared.

If you are a student standing at the edge of this profession, eager and uncertain, this is the story behind the textbooks. Patients do not arrive in bullet points. They bring fear, hope, trauma, complexity, and histories that refuse to fit neatly into algorithms. Medicine is not only science. It is humility, endurance, negotiation, accountability, and self-reflection. There are lessons here no lecture can teach. I learned many of them the long way.

This story is told through the mind of a rural doctor.

In small towns, medicine is not anonymous. Your patient may be your neighbor. The trauma victim may be your child's teacher. The cardiac arrest might happen in the grocery store aisle. Resources are limited, but responsibility is not. There is no army of subspecialists down the hall. No easy transfer when the roads close in a winter storm. There is only your team, your training, and the patient in front of you.

Rural medicine sharpens everything: the stakes, the relationships, the consequences. It reveals both the strength and fragility of the system. It is terrifying. It is humbling. It is beautiful.

There is good here: the newborn's first cry, the stroke patient who walks again, the farmer who grips your hand in gratitude. There is bad:

paperwork that steals time from patients, policies that make sense on paper but falter at the bedside, nights when you quietly question your limits. And there is ugly: preventable disease rooted in inequity, addiction unraveling families, moments when the system fails the very people it was built to serve.

All of it belongs in this story.

This is not a textbook. It is not a manifesto. It is a lived account of standing at the intersection of science and humanity long enough to see both its brilliance and its fractures.

I have seen it.

I have learned it.

I have lived it.

Now I invite you to see the world, just for a moment, through the mind of a rural doctor.

Then decide for yourself whether it scares you, amazes you, or leaves you in quiet awe of how much there is to learn.

Contents

The Man Himself: A Hero in Real Time

If I were asked to name the five people who shaped the architecture of my life, his name would not merely be on the list. It would rise to the top, etched there permanently.

He is the most extraordinary human being I have ever known.

An electrical engineer who became a cardiologist, he first mastered the invisible language of currents and circuits before dedicating himself to the even more complex circuitry of the human heart. Where others saw voltage and resistance, he saw harmony and precision. It feels almost inevitable that someone who understood electrical conduction would one day devote himself to the exquisite conduction system of the heart, mapping impulses not across wires, but across living tissue.

When he chose medicine, he did not simply practice it. He allowed it to take residence in his heart and bloodstream, indistinguishable from who he is.

For more than 50 years, he has listened to the quiet rhythms of humanity. He reads echocardiograms with architectural precision, rounds on the cardiology floor with steady purpose, sees patients in clinic with undiminished compassion, and teaches residents, fellows, and students as though each lecture might change a career. Often, it does.

He lives on a farm, not as nostalgia, but as discipline. On weekends, he returns to the soil, tending fields with the same devotion with which he tends ventricles and valves. There is something fitting about that. A man who restores circulation during the week cultivates life from the earth on Saturdays. Both require patience. Both demand humility. Both reward faith.

His mind is a cathedral of knowledge. Spend two hours with him and you leave altered, sharper and more awake to the world. He has mastered not only cardiology, but history, science in its broadest sense, politics, philosophy, and the quiet art of living well. Conversations with him do not feel like instruction. They feel like transformation.

What astonishes me most is that his curiosity has never dimmed. While many slow with time, he accelerates, especially into the frontier of artificial intelligence. He studies AI not as a spectator, but as a pioneer, exploring its role in imaging, diagnostics, and predictive cardiology. To hear him speak about machine learning algorithms alongside electrophysiology is to witness continuity, from electrical engineering to cardiac conduction to computational intelligence.

Technology does not intimidate him. It invigorates him. He adapts faster than most teenagers, not because he chases trends, but because he pursues improvement. He embraces innovation for one reason alone: to serve patients better.

The mark he has left on patients is immeasurable. Families kept whole. Milestones witnessed. Years restored. Across institutions and continents, he has traveled to teach, mentor, build programs, raise standards, and leave medicine better than he found it. His influence is not measured in titles or accolades, but in generations of physicians trained, systems strengthened, and lives extended.

Beyond the brilliance and legacy is the man himself.

Unconditional in his support. Steady in every storm. Present in the moments that mattered most. He offered guidance without ego, correction without humiliation, belief without hesitation. It is because of his example, mentorship, and relentless standard of excellence that I stand where I stand today.

Some heroes belong to history books.

Some belong to distant memory.

And then there are heroes you can call.

Heroes you can round with.

Heroes who answer your questions at midnight.

Heroes who farm at dawn, read echoes by noon, and study artificial intelligence by evening.

He is a hero in real time.

To dedicate words to him feels insufficient, because he has dedicated his life to something far greater than words: healing, teaching, cultivating both land and legacy. He has shown that intellect and humility can coexist, that strength and gentleness are not opposites, and that the true measure of a physician is not the length of a career, but the depth of impact.

If medicine lives in his heart, it is because his heart was always large enough to hold it.

This is my hero.

The Northwoods That Nearly Became Home

When I was in the final stretch of residency—those last, breathless months when the end feels both triumphant and terrifying—I received a call that seemed, at first, like destiny clearing its throat.

A recruiter from northern Wisconsin had been looking for someone exactly like me.

The position was in the Northwoods—a place spoken about in tones usually reserved for poetry. Dense forests stretching endlessly into the horizon. Lakes that caught the sky in their palms. Mornings wrapped in mist. Winters hushed beneath snow. A healthcare system in that region was preparing to build something new: a skilled nursing facility team led by a physician, supported by several advanced practice providers. The physician would oversee care across multiple nursing homes, bringing structure, continuity, and vision to a vulnerable population often overlooked.

They wanted me to lead it.

The idea struck a chord deep within me.

I have always had a love for geriatrics. During residency, we were fortunate—privileged, really—to train alongside a robust geriatrics fellowship program. We worked shoulder to shoulder with seasoned geriatricians whose wisdom seemed less learned than lived. They taught us that caring for the elderly was not simply about managing chronic disease; it was about preserving dignity. It was about navigating complexity—medical, emotional, social—with patience and reverence. They gave us a foundation that, I would argue, prepared us exceptionally well to care for this population.

So when this opportunity presented itself—my own team, my own program, dedicated entirely to the care of elders in their homes—it felt aligned. Purposeful. Almost providential.

The healthcare system invited me for an interview, and I decided to bring my wife and children along. If we were going to consider building a life somewhere, we would experience it together.

From the moment we arrived, we were enveloped in hospitality. They arranged a hotel, a rental car, meals—every detail thoughtfully handled. But what struck me most was not the comfort. It was the warmth.

The clinic visit felt less like an interview and more like a welcome. The providers greeted me not as competition or evaluation, but as a future colleague. There was an ease in their laughter. A sincerity in their handshakes. I could sense a culture of collaboration—of genuine friendship among physicians who respected one another.

The program director spoke passionately about life in the Northwoods. Most of the physicians, he told me, lived on acreages or along lakes. He showed me photographs of his own home—a beautiful property resting against shimmering water. In the summer, they boated and jet-skied beneath long golden sunsets. In the winter, the lake transformed into a frozen playground where families skated across its glassy surface. It was nature's rhythm, he said. Loud in its beauty, quiet in its pace.

A paradise for someone who loved stillness. For someone who wanted space.

One evening, they invited us to dinner at their golf club. The building overlooked rolling greens framed by forest, and the light that evening seemed to linger just for us. They had brought their families—spouses, children, laughter. My children found instant friends. My wife found easy conversation. There was no performance, no forced charm. These people were genuine in a way that is difficult to articulate. They were not selling a job. They were sharing a life.

That night, I tasted elk steak for the first time. It felt symbolic somehow—new, unfamiliar, rich with the flavor of a place that was not yet mine.

When we returned home, the offer came swiftly.

They liked what they saw.

And I liked what I felt.

But residency had given me more than clinical skills; it had given me mentors. Men and women who had invested in me—not just as a physician, but as a professional finding his trajectory. Whenever I faced a major decision, I turned to them.

This was no exception.

I shared the details. The role. The leadership. The beauty of the Northwoods. The culture. The team.

Almost unanimously, they advised against it.

Their reasoning was not dismissive of geriatrics—far from it. They understood my passion. But they urged me to think long-term. They encouraged me to begin my career practicing full-scope family medicine: inpatient and outpatient care, newborns to geriatrics, procedures, admissions, discharges—the entire spectrum.

"Build breadth first," they said. "Depth will come."

They worried that narrowing my focus too soon might limit my growth. That by stepping immediately into a geriatric-focused role, I would forgo the experience of managing the full continuum of care. They believed those early years were formative—that the muscle of clinical judgment strengthens most when stretched widely.

It was not the answer I wanted.

Turning down that offer was harder than I anticipated. I thought of the lake houses. The quiet winters. The elk steak. The laughter of our children mingling in a golf club dining room. I thought of the team I could have led, the nursing home residents whose stories I would have learned by heart.

But I trusted my mentors.

So I said no.

At the time, I'm not sure I fully grasped the wisdom in their advice. It felt like choosing uncertainty over comfort. Like walking away from something already tangible in favor of something undefined.

Yet looking back now, I believe it was the right decision.

Practicing full-scope medicine shaped me in ways I could not have predicted. Caring for newborns reminded me of beginnings. Managing complex hospital admissions sharpened my clinical acumen. Seeing patients across all ages deepened my adaptability. The rhythm of outpatient continuity visits grounded me in long-term relationships.

And geriatrics?

It never left me.

It remained woven into my practice—through nursing home coverage, through an aging rural population, through the privilege of walking alongside patients in the later chapters of their lives. I did not lose my love for geriatrics. If anything, it matured. It became informed by the broader experience of caring for families across generations.

In the end, that opportunity in the Northwoods was not a missed path. It was a crossroad. A reminder that sometimes the right decision is not the most enchanting one—but the one that stretches you.

The lakes, the snow, the elk steak—they remain a beautiful memory.

But the journey I chose gave me something just as profound: the confidence that comes from having seen it all, done it all, and grown through it all—before narrowing my focus.

And perhaps that, too, is its own kind of paradise.

From the Ditch to Destiny

Winter has a way of testing conviction.

I was a fourth-year medical student, dressed in my only interview suit, driving across southern Minnesota after what I thought had been a promising residency interview. It was late afternoon when I left—around 4 p.m.—the sky already fading into that gray Midwestern dusk. The snow had been light earlier, almost picturesque. The kind that makes a campus look charming and hopeful.

But as I merged onto I-90 west, the snow thickened. The wind picked up. The highway blurred into long white streaks. What had been manageable became treacherous.

I still remember the ramp.

One slight turn. One gentle correction. And then—nothing gentle at all. The tires lost their argument with physics. The car slid, slow at first, then helplessly, spinning into the ditch. Snow filled the windshield. Silence followed.

No injuries. Just adrenaline. And a thought that lodged itself deep in my mind:

Minnesota is not for me.

I climbed out of the ditch that evening convinced that whatever future I had, it would not involve winters like this.

Life, of course, has a sense of irony.

Four years later, at the end of residency, I found myself speaking with a recruiter from a large Midwestern healthcare system operating across Minnesota, South Dakota, Iowa, and North Dakota. She was refreshingly straightforward—no inflated promises, no sales pitch. Just honesty. She handed me a list of sites across the region and said, essentially, "Find where you belong."

I did my homework. I searched demographics, hospital data, school systems, community size. One town kept rising to the top: a community of about 13,000 people in southwest Minnesota.

Yes—Minnesota.

My wife and I visited. The people were warm. The clinicians were collaborative. It didn't feel transactional. It felt human. My children were comfortable. The schools seemed strong. The town had just enough life without losing its intimacy.

We said yes.

I began work there and quickly found what every young physician hopes for—support. Cohesive partners. A reliable hospital system. A steady patient base. It was stable and respectable.

But something felt incomplete.

My scope was narrower than I had imagined. Pediatrics were largely directed to subspecialized colleagues. I respected them deeply—but I missed the full spectrum of family medicine. I had trained broadly, and I wanted to practice broadly.

The administrative environment was different than I expected as well. The clinic director was an MBA—kind, polite, and numbers-driven. Productivity, margins, metrics. Necessary things, certainly. But I sometimes felt the tension between spreadsheets and stories. Between RVUs and real people. A patient is never just a line item—but it can feel that way in certain conversations.

Call was one in four nights and one weekend in four. On call nights, sleep was optional. Clinic the next morning was not. I remember days when I stared at the computer screen fighting gravity, reminding myself that the person in front of me deserved my best—even if I had been up most of the night.

The system itself was evolving—restructuring, reorganizing. Some changes were good. Others felt like change for the sake of change.

Then came the opportunity that altered everything.

About 25 miles down the road sat a smaller town—population 4,500. Their physician had traveled abroad and was unexpectedly unable to return due to visa complications. The clinic was left with APPs but no MD coverage. They needed help.

Our director asked if anyone would volunteer one day a week.

I raised my hand.

That first Friday, my schedule was blocked at my primary clinic. I drove out early, unsure what to expect.

The moment I walked through the doors, I felt something different.

The receptionist greeted me like an old friend. The nurse was prepared, organized, enthusiastic. The energy in the building was light but purposeful. Smaller space. Fewer exam rooms. But somehow… larger in spirit.

I saw nearly 20 patients that day—children with ear infections, elderly patients managing chronic disease, women's health concerns, acute complaints, routine follow-ups. The full spectrum.

It felt like family medicine again.

The clinic director wasn't even scheduled to work that day. Yet she showed up—with her two grandchildren in tow—just to introduce herself, to say thank you, to make me feel welcome. That small gesture said more than any contract ever could.

Throughout the day, staff members casually asked, "Are you transitioning here?"

"We'd love to have you."

"You fit here."

I drove home that evening with a feeling I hadn't felt in some time— professional fulfillment.

After a few more days helping there, it became clear: this wasn't just a temporary assist. This was alignment.

I spoke with the regional vice president—a thoughtful, approachable leader who respected physicians. I explained how I felt. She listened carefully, then smiled and said something simple and liberating:

"It doesn't matter to me which clinic you work at. They're both ours. I just want you where you'll thrive."

That sentence changed the trajectory of my career.

The transition was smooth. No territorial disputes. No political friction. Just professional respect.

Soon, I was splitting my time between two clinics about 10 miles apart—one existing MD at each site, supported by skilled APPs. We functioned as one team serving two communities. The scope was broad again. Pediatrics. Women's health. Geriatrics. Hospital work. The variety that makes family medicine dynamic and deeply meaningful.

Over time, the smaller town stopped feeling like a work location.

It became home.

Looking back, I think about that snowy ditch on I-90.

I had once sworn Minnesota off because of a winter storm.

Yet here I am—years later—having built a life, a career, and a leadership role in the very state I once doubted.

What changed?

Not the winters. They're still fierce.

But I learned that where you land isn't defined by the weather, the size of the town, or even the contract terms.

It's defined by people.

By culture.

By alignment of values.

By whether your work feels whole.

Sometimes the road spins you into a ditch before it guides you home.

And sometimes the place you feared becomes the place that shapes you—professionally, personally, and permanently.

If I had turned back that snowy evening and promised myself never to return, I would have missed the community that helped me grow, the colleagues who became friends, and the opportunity to practice medicine the way I had always envisioned.

Minnesota didn't just become where I worked.

It became where I belonged.

Earned, Not Assigned

Building a medical practice is not easy. It is not built in a day, a year, or even in the early stretch of enthusiasm that comes with a new diploma on the wall. It is built slowly—patient by patient, family by family, handshake by handshake.

I remember starting as a primary care provider in a small town of 4,500 people. A place where everyone knew everyone, where your name traveled faster than your CV ever could. We also had a satellite clinic 10 miles away, and I split my time 50–50 between the two. New physician. New face. No established panel. No long waiting list.

On most days, I saw five to seven patients. Occasionally ten. The schedule was light enough that I had time to read between visits, to dig deeper into guidelines, to refine my craft. It was, in many ways, a luxury. But it was also quiet—almost too quiet. I wasn't yet "someone's doctor." I was simply one of the doctors.

All of us cared for our own patients in the hospital, but with no panel of my own, my inpatient work was limited. I took 1-in-6 night call and 1-in-6 weekend community call, admitting for the entire community during those stretches. Otherwise, the hospital floors were mostly occupied by my partners' patients. I had two MD partners—one anchored at each clinic—and several APPs at both sites. Patients were scheduled with their designated provider, and if that provider was full, they were offered alternatives. I'm sure many chose someone familiar over the new guy.

Trust takes time. Especially in a small town.

In rural communities, patients don't just choose a clinician—they choose someone who may treat their children, their parents, and eventually themselves in a nursing home. They choose someone who will sit at kitchen tables, attend school events, and maybe even pray beside them in moments of crisis. You cannot rush that kind of trust. You earn it.

Slowly, gradually, my panel began to grow. A patient would return. Then bring a spouse. Then a neighbor. Word spreads quietly but powerfully in small-town America. Not through marketing campaigns, but through lived experiences.

Then change came.

My partner at the main clinic decided to move to Texas. I was pulled full-time to that clinic, no longer splitting my days between sites. Suddenly, the quiet days were gone. The practice took off. My schedule filled. Then overfilled. I went from reading between visits to racing between rooms.

Soon after, the partner at our satellite clinic retired. Overnight, I became the only MD between two clinics serving thousands of patients. We hired APPs to respond to the growing demand, and they were outstanding clinicians. But none of them did hospital work. That meant I became, by default, the hospitalist for all our patients from both clinics.

Full clinic days. Hospital rounds before and after. Admissions at night. Nursing home coverage for two facilities. Community call. Collaboration and supervision for APPs who relied on me for guidance and support.

Once simply another physician in the rotation, I grew into something far greater than a name on a schedule—I became foundational to the care of an entire community. What began with a handful of patients evolved into a practice built on trust, consistency, and unwavering presence. Over time, I was no longer just seeing patients; I was stewarding continuity of care for families who entrusted me with every stage of life.

As the sole physician between two clinics, I stepped into a role that extended beyond traditional boundaries—leading a fully integrated model of inpatient and outpatient medicine, coordinating care across hospital floors, clinic rooms, and nursing facilities. With the strength and partnership of our APPs and the steadfast support of administration, we shaped a resilient rural healthcare system—one designed not just to function, but to endure.

It was no longer about volume. It was about vision. About building something sustainable in a place where healthcare access depends on leadership willing to stay, to carry the weight, and to invest deeply in community. What started as a slow beginning became a platform for transformation—proving that in rural medicine, commitment can evolve into legacy.

It was busy. It was overwhelming at times. But it was also deeply meaningful.

Our affiliated hospital was supportive. Our administrators and clinic directors stood behind us. Our nursing teams were extraordinary— steady, loyal, and fiercely dedicated to our patients. In rural medicine, teamwork is not a buzzword. It is survival. It is sustainability.

Recruiting physicians to rural areas has never been easy. And this was no exception.

Years passed before we were finally able to recruit another physician to join me. He was finishing residency, full of promise, with hundreds of options before him. Like I once had. Like so many do.

He interviewed with us. He had a passion for rural health. But passion alone does not compete easily with urban opportunities, larger systems, and lighter call schedules.

I personally called him more than once. We spoke candidly—not just about workload, but about purpose. I told him about our patients. About the relationships. About the privilege of being there at the beginning of life and the end of life—and everywhere in between. I spoke highly of our nursing team, of our culture, of the meaning behind the work. I painted an honest picture: the challenges, the pace, the responsibility. But also the fulfillment.

I believe he saw himself here before he ever signed the contract.

He joined us.

And like me, he started slowly. Empty slots. A small trickle of patients. Introductions in exam rooms. Quiet days that test your patience and your confidence. He went through the same process of building trust—one family at a time.

In metropolitan areas, you can build a practice through visibility, systems, and scale. In small-town America, you build it through presence. Through consistency. Through showing up at 2 a.m. admissions. Through sitting longer in rooms when families are afraid. Through attending funerals. Through celebrating recoveries. Through being the steady physician year after year.

Building a practice here requires resilience. Patience. Perseverance. Humility. Endurance. Leadership. And above all, a genuine love for community.

It is not easy.

But when a patient looks at you and says, "You're my doctor," and they mean it—not because you were assigned to them, but because you earned it—that is something no fast start or big city contract can replicate.

In small-town America, a medical practice is not just built.

It is grown.

The Healing Power of Being Heard

One of the most underrated attributes of a good physician is the ability to truly listen. Not the kind of listening that waits impatiently for a pause, or plans the next question while the patient is still speaking—but the kind that allows silence, welcomes pauses, and respects the patient's need to complete a thought in their own time. The level of trust you build with your patients depends on it.

In reality, listening is not easy. It is surprisingly difficult to remain fully present for even 30 to 60 uninterrupted seconds while someone gathers their thoughts and tells their story. Our training pushes us toward efficiency, problem-solving, and rapid assessments. Yet, early in my practice, I discovered that intentional listening was one of the most powerful tools I could offer. When I applied it consistently, it transformed my patient relationships in ways no test or treatment ever could.

One patient in particular taught me this lesson more deeply than any other.

He was a retired pastor in his early 80s, living alone in a small apartment in town. He no longer drove and relied on public transportation for clinic visits and grocery shopping. On paper, he was just another elderly patient with a long problem list. In reality, he was thoughtful, articulate, deeply reflective, and—above all—someone who needed to be heard.

From the very first visit, it was clear that he came prepared. He arrived with pages of notes, a long list of questions, and a desire to understand every recommendation in detail. He did not like to be interrupted. He needed time to speak, to explain, to process out loud. I realized quickly that if I rushed him, or redirected the conversation too early, the connection would be lost.

So I did something simple but intentional: I listened.

I scheduled longer appointments for him. I allowed him the space to speak freely, without cutting him off. I followed his narrative before guiding the conversation back to medicine. And in doing so, something powerful happened—trust formed. Not the superficial kind, but the deep, relational trust that cannot be forced or rushed.

Over time, it became evident that this trust was unique. When I was unavailable, he never felt comfortable seeing another provider in our clinic. The staff often braced themselves when they saw his name on the schedule, knowing the visit would be long and complex. Other clinicians struggled to understand why connecting with him felt so difficult. But I knew the reason: he wasn't looking for answers alone—he was looking for a listener.

Every time he saw a specialist, he would schedule a follow-up appointment with me. He would bring their notes, their recommendations, and their plans, and ask me to help summarize them. More importantly, he wanted my thoughts. My reassurance. Sometimes even my approval. There were moments when I had no reason—or no position—to disagree with the specialist, but that wasn't the point. What mattered was that he trusted me enough to walk through those decisions with him.

As I came to know him better, I began to understand something deeper. Given his living situation and circumstances, he was likely lonely. Opportunities for meaningful conversation were rare. For him, the clinic was more than a medical stop—it was a place of human connection. A place where he felt seen, valued, and understood.

And that, too, is part of our job.

We are not here solely to treat physical ailments. We are here to support our patients in the ways they need us—emotionally, mentally, and sometimes simply by being present. Providing space for conversation, reflection, and connection can be just as therapeutic as any prescription.

Over the years, I have learned an incredible amount from my patients, and this patient was no exception. He shared his life story, his beliefs, his struggles, and his wisdom. I found his perspective educational on many levels—professionally and personally. He reminded me that medicine is as much about humanity as it is about science.

I eventually lost him to cancer.

But I will never forget him.

He left me with a lesson that continues to shape how I practice medicine: when you listen—truly listen—you do more than gather information. You build trust. You ease loneliness. You heal in ways that no chart, scan, or lab result ever could.

The Architecture of Trust

What do patients actually learn from how we run our clinic?

Not from our diplomas on the wall. Not from the ICD codes we enter. Not even from the diagnoses we make.

They learn from everything else.

They learn from the pause before the receptionist looks up. From the tone used when their name is called. From whether someone remembers they were anxious last time. Every clinic has a curriculum, and most of it is unspoken.

The education begins before the physician ever enters the room. It begins at the front desk. Is the greeting warm or merely efficient? Is eye contact made? Is the clipboard handed over with indifference or with guidance? Patients quickly decide: am I a number, or am I known? A hurried check-in teaches that health care is transactional. A human check-in teaches that this place sees me.

The medical assistant shapes more trust than we often realize. Do they rush through vitals, or do they ask what has been bothering you most? Do they sit, even briefly, at eye level? Do they convey that the physician has been informed and prepared? In those moments, patients learn whether their story matters. Trust is rarely built by a prescription. It is built by feeling heard before the physician ever enters.

We speak quickly. We think quickly. We move quickly. Patients do not. A clinic can unknowingly teach: keep up, or be left behind. Or it can teach: we will walk this with you. No patient remembers everything we say. Anxiety erases details. Illness narrows focus. Pain distracts memory. Written instructions are not a courtesy; they are essential. Clear summaries. Medication changes spelled out. Red flags explained. When we provide instructions both verbally and in writing, we communicate something profound: your understanding matters more than my efficiency.

The hidden curriculum does not end at checkout. It continues in how quickly phone calls are returned, in the tone of secure messages, in the clarity of refill policies, in whether abnormal labs trigger proactive outreach. When a patient waits days for a response, they learn that their concerns are small. When someone calls back the same day, even just to acknowledge receipt, they learn that they are being held in mind. Refill policies teach philosophy. They can feel like rigid barriers, or they can feel like structured systems delivered with compassion. Boundaries matter, but tone matters just as much. A system can be firm and still feel kind.

The patient experience is not segmented. It is global. Receptionist, medical assistant, nurse, physician, lab technician, checkout staff — to us these are roles; to the patient they are one organism. If one interaction is cold, the entire clinic feels cold. If one person goes above and beyond, the entire clinic feels extraordinary. Patients do not separate clinical care from customer service. They experience only care.

Every day, without realizing it, we teach our patients whether health is transactional or relational, whether their time matters, whether their questions are welcome, whether follow-up is their responsibility alone or a shared commitment. We may pride ourselves on diagnostic accuracy, but patients measure something different. They measure whether they feel safe. Whether they feel remembered. Whether they feel guided.

The follow-up call after a difficult diagnosis. The extra explanation when confusion is visible. The refill approved before a weekend so no one goes without. These are small acts, operationally minor, emotionally immense. They build a reservoir of trust that no single prescription can create.

The hidden curriculum of a clinic is always teaching. We cannot control every outcome, but we can control the atmosphere. We can design systems that quietly communicate: you are known, you are not alone, we are paying attention.

The only question is what we are choosing to teach.

The Weight of the White Coat

When a physician graduates from medical school, there is a ritual that feels symbolic but is, in truth, deeply practical. An oath is taken. Its origins trace back to Hippocrates around 400 BCE. The words have been revised many times to reflect modern ethics and social progress, yet the central commitments have endured.

The oath is less about tradition and more about restraint, character, and duty.

Medical professionalism rests on four enduring principles: beneficence, non-maleficence, autonomy, and justice. They are not abstract ideals; they are daily disciplines.

Beneficence asks the physician to act in the patient's best interest. This extends beyond diagnosing correctly or prescribing appropriately. It includes advocacy, thoughtful follow-through, intellectual curiosity, and emotional presence. It means using one's training, judgment, and influence to move a patient toward healing whenever possible. Even when cure is not achievable, relief of suffering and preservation of dignity remain obligations. Beneficence is an active posture toward good.

Closely linked is non-maleficence, often summarized as "first, do no harm." In practice, this principle is complex. Every intervention carries risk. Every medication has side effects. The discipline of medicine lies in balancing potential benefit against potential harm. It requires humility—the willingness to reconsider, to question whether an intervention is necessary, and to recognize the limits of one's knowledge. Harm is not only procedural or pharmacologic; it can be relational. Dismissiveness, haste, or poor communication can undermine trust as surely as a poorly chosen treatment.

Modern medicine also emphasizes autonomy. Historically, physicians often made decisions on behalf of patients. Contemporary professionalism rejects that model. The patient's body and life belong to the patient. The physician's role is to inform, guide, interpret evidence, and offer recommendations grounded in expertise. Shared decision-making respects the patient's values, priorities, and tolerance for risk. Professional maturity means accepting that a well-informed patient may choose differently than the physician would personally choose.

The final pillar, justice, extends professionalism beyond the individual encounter. Justice demands fairness. Care must not vary based on race, gender, age, socioeconomic status, political affiliation, religion, or lifestyle. Entering a clinical space requires leaving behind personal biases—both explicit and implicit. Every patient presents with a medical concern, not an identity to be judged. Justice reflects the ethical equivalent of the Golden Rule: provide the same standard of care you would expect for your own family.

Threaded through all four principles are confidentiality and integrity. Patients disclose intimate details because they trust the profession. That trust is fragile. Safeguarding privacy, admitting errors, disclosing conflicts of interest, and committing to lifelong learning are not optional virtues; they sustain the moral credibility of medicine.

Professionalism is tested less in moments of triumph and more in moments of strain—fatigue, uncertainty, disagreement, or poor outcomes. It is easy to be principled when cases are straightforward. The measure of character appears when they are not.

In the end, the oath is not a ceremonial artifact. It is a framework for daily conduct. Do no harm. Act for good. Respect patient choice. Treat all fairly. These principles are simple to state and lifelong to master.

Medicine remains, at its core, a moral endeavor carried out through scientific means.

Beyond Titles: A Shared Oath

Few topics in modern medicine spark as much emotion as the role of advanced practice providers—nurse practitioners and physician assistants, often referred to as APPs. In some states, they practice independently. In others, they work under varying degrees of physician supervision. For some physicians, this evolution has been uncomfortable. For others, it has been transformative. For all of us, it has been unavoidable.

To understand the tension, you have to understand the training.

The road to becoming a physician is long and demanding. Take Family Medicine, for example: four years of college, four years of medical school, and three years of residency—an intense, immersive apprenticeship in real-world medicine. Nights. Weekends. Holidays. ICU rotations. Labor and delivery. Pediatrics. Inpatient medicine. Emergency care. Outpatient continuity clinic.

By the time a family physician graduates, they have delivered at least 40 babies and managed approximately 1,600 patients in clinic under direct supervision. They have been stretched, tested, humbled, and refined. The breadth is intentional. The repetition is deliberate. The responsibility is heavy.

There is no shortcut to that.

APPs follow a different path. Their education, while rigorous in its own right, is shorter and more focused. It does not include the same depth in anatomy, physiology, pathology, and pharmacology, nor does it require a multi-year residency across multiple specialties and hospital services. Most enter practice directly after completing their formal training. For some physicians, this contrast raises concern. The question is not about intelligence or dedication—it is about equivalency of preparation and the responsibilities that follow.

And yet, the story does not end there.

Because healthcare in America does not exist in theory. It exists in rural towns, busy clinics, emergency rooms at 2 a.m., and communities where access is fragile. We simply do not have enough physicians—especially in rural areas. Patients still need care. Chronic diseases still progress. Babies still need to be delivered. Emergencies still walk through the door.

APPs have become essential to meeting that need.

Economics plays a role. A physician may cost two to three times as much as an APP. Health systems, under pressure to remain financially viable, have adapted. Many have adopted collaborative care models where physicians and APPs work together—sharing panels, dividing responsibilities, supporting one another in clinic and specialty services. When structured thoughtfully, these models work remarkably well.

Over time, most physicians—including many who were once skeptical—have come to recognize this reality. APPs are not a replacement for physicians. They are not a shortcut to becoming one. They are a different profession with a different training pathway, serving a critical role in a strained system.

Personally, I view APPs as indispensable. Nearly every APP I have worked with has understood their scope of practice and their limits. That self-awareness is the foundation of safe medicine. I believe there should always be a level of support and physician collaboration available—not as a constraint, but as a safeguard and a resource. Medicine is too complex for isolation.

What has impressed me most is what happens over time. APPs who practice for years within a specific specialty develop extraordinary proficiency. Repetition sharpens skill. Pattern recognition deepens. Confidence grows. In their focused areas, many become remarkably adept—sometimes approaching the practical fluency of their physician counterparts within that defined scope.

I have been fortunate. The APPs I have worked alongside have been exceptional—clinically capable, thoughtful, compassionate. Our professional relationships have grown into something more meaningful: trust, respect, camaraderie. I would confidently entrust any of them with my own care or that of my family. That is not a statement I make lightly.

This debate is not about hierarchy. It is about responsibility. It is about training differences, patient safety, access to care, and the realities of modern healthcare. It is also about humility—the recognition that no one clinician can carry the entire system alone.

Medicine works best as a team sport.

Physicians bring the depth and breadth forged through years of structured training. APPs bring skill, adaptability, and critical access— especially where physicians are scarce. Together, when aligned by mutual respect and clear roles, they create something stronger than either could alone.

In the end, the question is not whether APPs belong in our healthcare system.

They are already here.

The real question is whether we choose to build a system defined by competition—or one strengthened by collaboration. From my experience, the answer is clear.

Where Many Hands Hold One Life

Most people see medicine as a moment.

A knock on a door.

A stethoscope on a chest.

A prescription sent to a pharmacy.

A discharge paper folded into a purse or jacket pocket.

What they do not see is the orchestra.

Before a single pill reaches a bedside, it pauses in the careful hands of a pharmacist — a quiet guardian asking invisible questions. Is the kidney strong enough? Is the dose too bold? Does this drug quarrel with another? Is there an allergy whispered somewhere in the chart? The medication waits until the answer is safe.

In clinics and emergency rooms, prescriptions travel through unseen circuits of review. If something feels off, a phone rings. A conversation happens. A correction is made. Safety is rarely dramatic. It is deliberate.

I tell our students there is no room for error in medicine. The sky does not forgive a pilot's inattention. Gravity is impartial. So we build checklists. We build redundancies. We build systems that assume we are human — and therefore capable of missing something.

Because we are human.

Errors still happen. Not from indifference, but from complexity. From fatigue. From the sheer weight of variables that accompany every patient. The answer has never been perfection. The answer has been partnership.

Advanced practice providers do not stand alone. They work in rhythm with collaborating physicians. Orders are reviewed. Notes are co-signed. Plans are discussed before they are finalized. Another perspective is invited before it is required. A second set of eyes is not a sign of weakness — it is a safeguard. It is how we honor the gravity of what we do.

I believe deeply in second opinions. When an illness lingers without clarity, when a diagnosis feels just out of reach, when progress stalls and questions multiply — a fresh mind can illuminate what familiarity may have quietly dimmed. Not because someone has failed, but because medicine is complex. Because patients are complex. Because humility protects what confidence alone cannot.

In medicine, certainty should never become isolation. The safest care is rarely built by one voice. It is shaped in dialogue — refined, questioned, strengthened — until the plan is not just reasonable, but resilient.

Every morning, at bedsides bathed in early light or in quiet conference rooms before the day surges forward, a small circle forms. Five. Sometimes eight. A physician. A nurse. A pharmacist. A social worker. A care coordinator. A physical therapist. An occupational therapist. A dietitian. Each carries a different lens. Each holds a different piece of the same life.

We do not only review lab values and imaging. We ask quieter questions.

Who waits at home?

Are there stairs?

Is there food in the refrigerator?

Will they remember their medications?

Can they afford them?

Who will drive them to follow-up?

Safe discharge is not a signature. It is a promise.

It may mean a home safety evaluation to prevent the fall that would undo everything. It may mean a walker fitted just right, a shower chair placed carefully, a hospital bed delivered before sunset. It may mean medications organized into bubble packs by a trusted local pharmacist. A reminder system blinking softly on a kitchen counter. Home health nurses. Home physical therapy. A home health aide. County social work. Community transit. Small structures that hold up fragile independence.

Especially for our elders, success after hospitalization is built on details that never make the discharge summary.

We pause before procedures and confirm the right patient, the right site, the right plan. We reconcile medications line by line. We standardize handoffs so that information does not dissolve between the tired and the rested. We study near-misses not to punish, but to understand. Where did the net thin? Where can we weave it tighter?

There is no applause for the mistake that never happens.

No headline for the fall prevented.

No ceremony for the readmission avoided.

No recognition for the phone call that caught a dangerous dose in time.

Yet this is the work.

And when harm does occur, we do not look away. We speak honestly. We take responsibility. We learn. We rebuild. We add another checkpoint. We strengthen the bridge for the next person who must cross it.

Medicine is not a solo act. It is a constellation of careful minds orbiting a single goal: safety.

So when you see one clinician in a room, know that there are many behind that moment. An unseen circle, every morning, leaning over charts and lives with equal gravity. Asking again and again, in different voices but with the same intention:

Is this safe?

Is this right?

Have we missed anything?

Safety in medicine is not assumed.

It is constructed — quietly, collaboratively, and with humility —

one patient, one checkpoint, one careful decision at a time.

The Work of Hands and Hope

Musculoskeletal pain is the quiet rhythm of everyday medicine.

It slips into clinic without announcement—an aching shoulder, a swollen knee, a back that "just hasn't been right," a runner with a stress fracture, a warehouse worker with carpal tunnel, a farmer with chronic hip pain that he has ignored for months. There doesn't go a day without it. It is ordinary. Constant. Human.

For those still in residency, here is something I have learned: learn this well.

Not because it is glamorous. Not because it wins awards.

But because it will fill your days.

Master the shoulder exam. Respect the knee. Understand the spine. Learn to inject with confidence and precision. Spend time with sports medicine if you can. Watch how they examine, how they think, how they treat function—not just pathology. I was fortunate to train alongside a sports medicine fellowship and even carved out extra time to deepen those skills. That experience still echoes in my practice.

But the deeper lesson was not about injections or maneuvers.

It was about rehabilitation.

The patient with stubborn lateral epicondylitis who doesn't improve with rest and NSAIDs—therapy changes the trajectory.

The person with chronic low back pain who has lost strength and trust in their body—rehab rebuilds both.

The woman with cervical radiculopathy—gentle traction and guided exercises relieve what pills never could.

The older adult who falls—gait training restores stability and independence.

The patient with Parkinson's disease—structured therapy slows functional decline.

The patient with vertigo—vestibular rehab gives back balance, literally and figuratively.

Over time, you begin to realize something profound: we diagnose, but they restore.

I have said this many times, and it remains true:

I don't think I can practice medicine without therapy.

That is not exaggeration. It is lived experience.

When I walk into clinic or the hospital, I know that behind many of my best outcomes stands a physical therapist, an occupational therapist, a rehabilitation team translating medical plans into movement, strength, coordination, and confidence. They sit with patients through repetition and frustration. They witness progress in millimeters that become miles.

Medicine without rehab would feel incomplete—like identifying the problem without walking the patient toward recovery.

To my therapy colleagues: your work is steady, skilled, and transformative. You do not just treat joints and muscles. You restore dignity, mobility, and hope. I am grateful for you every single day.

Care Without Condition

A patient comes in before an election and asks, "How should I vote?"

You pause and respond, "That's the last thing I can help you with. That's your personal choice. I'm here for your medical care."

It seems like a simple exchange, but it touches on a deeper issue: what role, if any, should a physician's political beliefs play in medical practice?

Physicians are citizens. We live in the same communities as our patients. We vote, hold opinions, and care about issues that shape society. Expecting physicians to have no political beliefs is unrealistic. The more meaningful question is whether those beliefs influence how we care for patients.

Some clinicians argue that their personal views do not affect their practice. They treat every patient the same, regardless of political affiliation, background, or ideology. Others worry that strong political convictions—like any strong belief—can subtly influence judgment, communication style, or the framing of options, particularly in areas that intersect with public debate.

The exam room, however, is not a political space. It is a clinical one. The physician's authority in that room is grounded in medical knowledge, experience, and a commitment to patient welfare—not in political opinion. When a patient asks for voting advice, setting a respectful boundary protects the integrity of the therapeutic relationship. It keeps the focus where it belongs: on the patient's health.

Patients come from across the political spectrum. In a single clinic day, a physician may care for individuals who hold very different views on social and political issues. The strength of medicine as a profession lies in its ability to provide consistent, equitable care regardless of those differences. The commitment to treat each person with dignity and without discrimination is foundational. It is embedded in our training, our ethical codes, and the oath we take.

The greater risk is not that physicians have beliefs, but that they lack self-awareness about how those beliefs may shape their interactions. Strong convictions—political, religious, or cultural—can influence tone, assumptions, and counseling if left unexamined. Professional maturity requires reflection. It requires asking: "Am I presenting options neutrally? Am I listening openly? Am I respecting this patient's values even when they differ from my own?"

Some argue that physicians should strive to be entirely apolitical, similar to judges. In practice, complete neutrality in personal belief is neither achievable nor necessary. What is necessary is professional discipline. The patient's values guide decision-making. The physician provides evidence-based recommendations, outlines risks and benefits, and supports informed choices. Personal ideology should not determine access, quality, or compassion.

Ultimately, the core obligation is clear: care for the patient in front of you—regardless of class, political identity, socioeconomic status, religion, or background. The trust patients place in physicians depends on their confidence that they will be treated fairly and respectfully.

The debate about politics in medicine will continue. What remains steady is the profession's central promise. In the exam room, the patient comes first.

One Size Does Not Fit All: The Art and Science of Individualized Care

One size does not fit all in medicine. Clinical trials give us averages. Guidelines give us structure. But no patient walks into our exam room as an average.

Evidence-based medicine was never meant to be "cookbook" medicine. It was meant to combine the best available evidence with clinical judgment and, just as importantly, the patient's own values and circumstances. The data tell us what works for most people. Our job is to decide what will work for this person.

Two patients can share the same diagnosis, the same labs, and the same imaging—and respond very differently to the same treatment. Biology varies. Life circumstances vary. Motivation varies. Support systems vary. Risk tolerance varies. If we ignore those differences, we may follow the guideline perfectly and still fail the patient.

There is a difference between treating hypertension and treating Mrs. Johnson's hypertension. One patient fears medications because of past side effects. Another wants the most aggressive therapy possible after watching a parent suffer a stroke. One struggles with cost. Another struggles with complexity. Adjusting therapy to their realities is not compromising care; it is delivering better care.

We often quote the golden rule: treat others the way you want to be treated. In medicine, a higher standard applies—treat people the way they want to be treated. Some patients want detailed data and shared decision-making. Others want clear direction. Some need reassurance. Others need urgency. The art lies in adjusting ourselves—our tone, our pace, our plan—to meet them where they are.

When patients feel understood, trust grows. When trust grows, adherence improves. When adherence improves, outcomes improve.

Compliance is rarely about stubbornness; it is often about misalignment between the plan we create and the life they live.

Individualized care does not mean abandoning standards. It means applying them wisely. Protocols provide safety. Evidence provides direction. Experience provides judgment. The patient provides context. The skill of the physician is blending all four.

Knowing your patients—professionally and personally—changes everything. When we put ourselves in their shoes and tailor care to who they are, not just what they have, we practice medicine at its highest level. One size does not fit all. And it never should.

Two Voices in Medicine: The Space Between Science and Choice

When I was a resident, I began to notice something that wasn't written in any textbook.

It lived in the exam room.

There seemed to be two ways physicians spoke when it came time to recommend something. Two tones. Two postures. Two quiet philosophies of care.

Some would sit down and speak plainly.

"This is what the guidelines recommend. Here are the benefits. Here are the risks. This is why I suggest it."

They were clear. Direct. Respectful of autonomy. If the patient declined, they might explore the reason briefly. And if the answer remained no, they would nod, document, and move on. The relationship mattered more than winning the moment. There would be another visit, another chance.

Others leaned in differently.

They asked more questions. They listened for hesitation. They returned to the topic again, sometimes twice in the same visit. If a patient declined a flu vaccine, they might re-enter the room themselves and say gently, "Let's talk about this one more time." They believed that if they found the right angle, the right story, the right connection, they might change a mind — and perhaps change a life.

As residents, we never quite knew which style we were supposed to adopt. One attending valued concise recommendations and forward movement. Another expected persistence and proof that we could motivate. Depending on the week, the definition of a "good job" shifted.

Neither approach was wrong. Both were rooted in care.

Over time, something else became clear: even the most measured physician carries quiet passions.

One lingers over adolescent safety — seat belts, helmets, distracted driving — because they have seen the aftermath of a preventable crash. Another slows down when discussing cancer screening, unwilling to miss something that could have been caught early. Someone else returns, again and again, to vaccines.

We tell ourselves we are neutral messengers of science. But we are human. What we have witnessed shapes how long we stay in the room. It shapes how hard we try.

And then there are the guidelines.

Patients often imagine a single, unified rulebook behind every recommendation. In reality, medicine speaks in many voices. Primary care physicians often look to the U.S. Preventive Services Task Force. Specialists may look to their own professional societies. These groups examine the same data but sometimes arrive at different conclusions — different ages to begin screening, different thresholds for treatment, different assessments of risk and benefit.

The public sees contradiction.

Physicians see interpretation.

Add to that another truth: the rules change. Over the past decade and a half, screening ages have shifted. Blood pressure targets have moved. Cholesterol management has been rewritten. Therapies once encouraged are now discouraged; practices once dismissed have found new footing. What we said confidently ten years ago may not hold today.

This is not instability. It is science breathing. It is evidence evolving. But from the outside, it can feel unsettling.

"Doctor, last time you said something different."

Yes. Because last time, the data was different.

Patients also ask why their primary physician says one thing while their specialist says another. Often, both are right within their frameworks. A specialist sees the worst outcomes of a specific disease and may lean toward aggressive prevention. A generalist sees the broader population — the harms of overtesting, the anxiety of false positives, the cost of overtreatment. Perspective influences emphasis.

What looks like disagreement is often nuance.

Behind every recommendation is a balancing act: evidence, risk, patient values, time constraints, lived experience. In a twenty-minute visit, we try to reconcile them all.

How long should we stay with a patient who says no? When does persistence become pressure? When does respect for autonomy become avoidance of a hard conversation? There is no universal answer. Each physician develops a threshold — a sense of which hills are worth standing on and which can wait.

With time, many of us settle somewhere between the two styles we observed in training. We make clear recommendations. We explain the reasoning. We leave space for choice. Sometimes we revisit. Sometimes we let it rest. And sometimes, when a topic carries particular weight — shaped by evidence or by memory — we lean in a little more.

Medicine is not a script delivered from certainty. It is a conversation held in uncertainty, guided by imperfect but improving knowledge.

If your doctors sound different from one another, it is not always because one is careless. It is often because medicine is complex, because guidelines are not uniform, because evidence shifts, because perspective matters.

Inside the exam room, we are not flipping coins. We are navigating a moving landscape, trying to honor both science and the person sitting in front of us.

There are not truly two camps — preaching and recommending — but a spectrum of voices shaped by data, experience, and conscience. Most of us move along that spectrum, sometimes firm, sometimes gentle, always hoping that what we offer is not just correct, but compassionate.

And often, we continue the conversation — not because we need to win, but because we care enough to try.

Where Medicine Feels Human Again: The Calling of Rural Practice

The practice of medicine is sacred no matter where it is done. Whether in a bustling academic center or a small community hospital, the responsibility and privilege of caring for another human being never changes. Yet, for me, medicine practiced in a rural setting carries a unique depth of meaning and fulfillment that is hard to replicate elsewhere.

One of the greatest joys of rural medicine is the breadth of practice it allows. In rural settings, physicians are often called upon to be more than just one thing. You are a clinician, a problem-solver, an emergency responder, a hospitalist, and often a trusted advisor. That wide scope brings a deep sense of professional satisfaction. You get to use every bit of what you learned during training—the knowledge, the procedures, the clinical judgment—and you continue to grow because your work demands it. For physicians who value versatility and mastery across disciplines, rural medicine is not a limitation; it is an invitation.

The distance from specialists and tertiary care centers undeniably places strain on rural facilities and providers. But within that challenge lies one of rural medicine's greatest strengths: innovation born of necessity. Limited resources force you to think creatively, to problem-solve thoughtfully, and to make the absolute best use of what you have. You learn to practice medicine with intention and efficiency. Decisions matter. Judgment matters. And when you deliver excellent care despite constraints, the reward is profound. There is something deeply gratifying about knowing that your skills and leadership directly shape outcomes in a setting where every resource counts.

Yes, rural practice can be demanding. The expectations are broad, and the workload can be heavy. You may find yourself moving between clinic, inpatient floors, and the emergency department, sometimes all in the same day. There are moments when you feel stretched. But that same intensity is what makes the work meaningful. You are not just another physician in a large system—you are essential. Your presence matters. Your absence is felt. That sense of purpose fuels resilience and pride in your work.

Rural life itself offers a quieter, more grounded rhythm. There is no traffic stealing hours from your day. You can get to work and back home quickly, reclaiming precious time for family, rest, and reflection. The quietness, the open spaces, and the slower pace bring a sense of balance that is increasingly rare in modern medicine. These are not small things—they are quality-of-life gifts that sustain longevity in practice.

Perhaps the most powerful aspect of rural medicine is the depth of relationships it fosters. In rural communities, you truly know your patients. You see them not just in exam rooms but in grocery stores, at school events, and at community gatherings. Your children go to school with their children. You know their families, their struggles, their values, and their histories. Over time, medicine becomes more than transactional—it becomes relational.

Trust grows naturally in these settings. Patients trust you not just because of your credentials, but because they know you as a person. They know you are invested in their lives and their community. That mutual trust strengthens care in ways no protocol or technology ever could. Healing becomes a shared journey rather than a series of isolated encounters.

Rural medicine also offers a rare opportunity to lead and shape healthcare delivery. In smaller systems, physicians often have a direct voice in decision-making, quality improvement, and program development. You can see the impact of your ideas quickly and tangibly. Change is not buried under layers of bureaucracy—it is visible, immediate, and meaningful.

There is also a deep sense of gratitude in rural communities. Patients appreciate your presence, your effort, and your commitment. They understand the sacrifices required to practice in a rural setting, and they do not take it for granted. That gratitude is humbling and energizing, reminding you why you chose medicine in the first place.

Rural medicine strips healthcare down to its core: service, responsibility, and human connection. It challenges you, stretches you, and sometimes exhausts you—but it also rewards you in ways that go far beyond productivity metrics or academic titles.

In rural health, you are not just practicing medicine.

You are part of the community.

You are trusted.

You are needed.

And in that space, medicine feels deeply human again.

That is why I love rural health.

Keepers of the Calling: They Keep the Door Open

In towns scattered across the Midwest—places with one stoplight, a water tower, and a café where everyone knows everyone—there is a quiet tradition that almost no one outside medicine sees.

Community physicians volunteer to teach.

No requirement.

No real financial incentive.

No reduction in workload.

Just a name added to a list sent to a medical school each year:

"Yes, I'll take a student."

Most of these towns have populations between 2,000 and 15,000. The doctors who practice there are not insulated by layers of residents or fellows. They carry the pager themselves. They round on their own patients. They show up when the ambulance tones drop at 2 a.m.

And still, they say yes to teaching.

Medical schools across the Midwest deliberately send students into these communities. Rural rotations are not accidental; they are formative. Students are required to leave academic centers and step into real towns where medicine is not compartmentalized. In those places, a student does not compete for experience.

A student participates.

That participation exists because preceptors make room for it.

They rearrange clinic schedules. They accept that the day will move slower. They allow a student to examine first, to present first, to attempt procedures under watchful eyes. They absorb the inefficiency without complaint. Teaching costs time. Time costs money. In small practices, margins are not generous.

Yet every year, they volunteer again.

When the list of available sites was distributed to our class, it contained more than one hundred names. Next to many of them were handwritten notes: housing provided, meals included, stipend available. These were not institutional dormitories or funded academic housing arrangements. These were homes. Spare bedrooms. Finished basements. Hospital call rooms converted for temporary use.

The generosity was assumed, not advertised.

One physician in a college town of 5,000 took a student into his already full professional life. Fifteen miles away, in a farming town of 900, he ran a satellite clinic where he knew nearly every patient by name. He saw newborns and grandparents in the same morning. He rounded in the hospital. He covered the emergency room. And during football season, he still made time to gather with friends at the local bar, where he was not "Doctor" so much as neighbor.

When a student arrived, the town noticed. The local paper asked for an interview. Not because the student was remarkable, but because the presence of a learner meant something hopeful: the next generation was paying attention.

Another physician—his son—practiced in a town of 1,200. His scope was even broader. He performed endoscopies and colonoscopies. Delivered babies. Performed C-sections. Managed admissions. Covered emergencies. There were no specialists down the hall. If something needed to be done, he either did it or arranged the transfer himself.

And still, he took students.

Hosting a learner is not merely allowing shadowing. It is opening the inner workings of a life. It is answering questions between patients. It is staying current enough to teach. It is accepting scrutiny with humility.

A student's presence quietly raises the standard of everyone in the building. Nurses explain more carefully. Physicians articulate reasoning they might otherwise carry silently. The entire practice sharpens.

The sacrifices are rarely visible.

One preceptor noticed a student's car struggling as it rolled into town. With a single phone call, he arranged for his personal mechanic to repair it. No invoice was handed over. No awkward conversation followed. It was simply handled. In rural communities, relationships precede transactions.

Another time, housing meant a room in a hospital basement—dim, largely unused, directly across from the morgue. Not glamorous. Not curated for comfort. But offered sincerely. What mattered was not luxury; it was access. Proximity to patients. Proximity to responsibility. Proximity to the unfiltered reality of medicine.

Preceptors understand something that cannot be taught in lecture halls: comfort does not form physicians. Exposure does.

They bring students along when ambulance tones drop for an unresponsive patient. They allow them to attempt procedures under supervision. They let them feel the weight of chest compressions that do not restore a pulse. They model composure when forty minutes of resuscitation ends in silence.

And afterward, they teach the lesson that matters most: effort and excellence are required, even when outcomes are not guaranteed.

They do this not for recognition, but for continuity.

When these physicians were students, someone opened a door for them. Someone slowed down. Someone answered questions patiently. The tradition was handed to them without ceremony, and they accepted the responsibility to pass it forward.

It is generational stewardship.

Years later, those relationships often endure. Holiday cards are exchanged. Former students become colleagues. Sometimes, in seasons of crisis, a preceptor will quietly search for a former student, drive across counties, and knock on the door of the clinic where that student now practices—just to check in.

That is not part of any curriculum requirement.

That is character.

The public rarely sees this architecture beneath medical education—the spare bedrooms offered without charge, the meals shared, the repaired cars, the financial inefficiencies accepted, the intellectual vulnerability of allowing a student to ask, "Why?"

But this is how physicians are truly formed.

Not solely in tertiary hospitals.

Not exclusively through exams and evaluations.

But in exam rooms in towns of 900 people.

In operating rooms where family doctors perform procedures because no one else is coming.

In emergency departments where the community doctor carries the code pager personally.

These preceptors do more than teach medicine.

They model ownership. Accountability. Humility. Breadth. Community trust.

They show that a physician is not defined by subspecialty prestige or institutional affiliation, but by presence—by being the one who stays when everyone else transfers out.

Now, as another generation of students rotates through rural towns, the tradition continues. Community physicians still add their names to the list.

They still rearrange schedules.

They still open homes.

They still absorb the cost.

Quietly.

Deliberately.

Faithfully.

The system depends on them more than it acknowledges.

They are the ones who keep the door open.

Staying, So the Doors Stay Open

Across America, the map is dotted with small hospitals—some weathered by time, some newly renovated but equally fragile—standing at the edge of cornfields, mountains, plains, and coastal towns. Fewer of them remain independent now. Each year, more close their doors, trim services, or join the protective umbrella of a larger system in order to survive.

Rural hospitals struggle in ways that are both visible and unseen. Reimbursement margins are thin. Patient volumes fluctuate with seasons and local industry. A single departure—a surgeon, a family physician, a CRNA—can ripple through the entire community. Recruiting talent to a small town is not just about compensation; it is about schools, spousal employment, childcare, and call schedules that stretch a limited workforce. Rising supply costs, regulatory demands, aging infrastructure, and payer mix realities weigh heavily.

Financial viability is not theoretical here—it is existential.

Some hospitals merge into large healthcare systems and gain the stability of scale: stronger purchasing power, broader specialty access, capital for technology, shared compliance infrastructure, and deeper administrative support. There is safety in size. There is efficiency in centralization. For many communities, this partnership preserves access that might otherwise disappear.

But something shifts when a hospital becomes part of a larger machine. Decisions are often made at a corporate level and cascade downward. Strategy aligns across regions. Standardization replaces improvisation. There are advantages—consistency, resources, shared expertise—but there is also distance. The voice of the individual employee may feel quieter in the echo of a vast organization.

In smaller independent hospitals, decisions are made locally. The board members are neighbors. Leadership walks the same hallways as environmental services. Strategy is shaped not only by spreadsheets but by faces. Employees often find they have a voice—not just in policy, but in culture. Change can happen quickly. Innovation can be personal. Accountability is close and human.

There are trade-offs. Independence demands resilience. It requires long nights balancing budgets, difficult service-line decisions, and constant recruitment efforts. It asks nurses to pick up extra shifts when staffing is tight. It asks administrators to stretch every dollar. It asks leaders to carry uncertainty quietly.

And yet—many remain.

This is for them.

For the receptionist who greets each morning with a steady smile, offering warmth before the day has fully begun. For the administrative professional behind a closed office door long after sunset, still reconciling numbers to keep the doors open one more year. For the staff member arranging childcare through family favors, determined not to leave colleagues short-handed.

For environmental services and housekeeping teams whose unseen diligence protects every patient. For cafeteria staff who nourish bodies and spirits alike, handing over trays and coffee with a kindness that refuels more than hunger.

For nurses working mandated overtime, covering for a colleague with a sick child, charting past midnight, returning again at dawn. Selflessness in real time.

For laboratory technicians, radiology technologists, maintenance crews, pharmacists, physicians, therapists, billing staff—the entire quiet ecosystem that sustains a community's access to care.

Independent rural hospitals are not simply buildings. They are acts of collective will.

They represent a community's refusal to surrender local care. They are sustained by people who believe that proximity matters—that healing close to home is worth fighting for. That a hospital is not just an access point in a network, but a heartbeat in a town.

There is nothing inherently wrong with large systems. They save hospitals. They stabilize regions. They deliver excellence at scale.

But there is something profoundly moving about those still standing independently—balancing on narrow margins, tightening belts, trimming where they must, innovating where they can—so that when an ambulance arrives at 2 a.m., the lights are on.

This is a dedication to those who show up anyway.

To those who serve not for recognition, but for community.

To those whose dedication is not loud, but unwavering.

In a time of consolidation, they remain—

steadfast, local, human—

holding the line for their neighbors.

Guardians of the Gentle Season

Skilled nursing facilities occupy a sacred space in medicine. They are the in-between—the bridge from hospital to home, from crisis to stability, from uncertainty to routine. For many patients, they become more than facilities; they become home. A place where healing continues at a gentler pace, where dignity is protected, and where presence matters as much as prescriptions.

In our community, there were two SNFs—one in town and another 10 miles away. One building housed up to 70 residents, and our system cared for approximately half of them. The second facility cared for up to 60 residents, and our practice managed nearly 90% of their care. The work was deeply rooted in geriatrics. These were not brief encounters, but long chapters—stories unfolding over seasons, relationships built over time.

Leadership became part of that journey. Serving as Medical Director for one facility, and later stepping in to guide another SNF an hour away after it lost its director, revealed how much thoughtful structure supports compassionate care. Policies were refined. Antibiotic stewardship strengthened. Care transitions were streamlined. Behind every regulation and protocol was a simple goal: protect the resident.

The heart of these facilities, however, is the staff. Nurses, CRNAs, therapists, pharmacists, aides—each plays a critical role. Residents often rely entirely on caregivers for activities of daily living: bathing, toileting, transfers, fall precautions, pressure injury prevention, medication management. In these settings, small details matter enormously. A subtle change in mentation. A new cough. A decrease in appetite. Vigilance is constant.

Yet staffing shortages and financial constraints weigh heavily on the system. When staffing thins, the impact is immediate and profound—higher risk of falls, delayed care, avoidable hospital transfers, emotional strain for families, moral strain for caregivers. In rural communities especially, these facilities are lifelines. Without them, hospitals cannot discharge safely, families must travel far from home, and fragile patients lose the comfort of familiarity. Rural SNFs are not conveniences; they are pillars holding up the entire continuum of care.

Recently, I learned the term SNFist—a physician dedicated to the care of nursing facility residents. The word may be new, but the calling is not. I have been proud to call myself a SNFist for many years. It is a role that requires patience, attentiveness, and respect for the slow rhythm of geriatric medicine.

As a hospitalist, there is reassurance in knowing that when a patient cannot safely return home, there is a place prepared to receive them— a team ready to continue the work. Skilled nursing facilities are where recovery is nurtured, where comfort is prioritized, where community endures even in frailty.

Their sustainability is essential. They are homes for elders, partners to hospitals, anchors for rural towns, and guardians of dignity. In the quiet work done within their walls lies something profoundly important: the steady, faithful care of those who once cared for us.

Where the House Becomes Sacred: The Quiet Grace of a Doctor at the Bedside

There is something timeless about the image of a physician at a patient's bedside—not in a hospital room humming with monitors, but in a quiet home. The old leather bag. The knock at the door. The quiet exchange in a familiar living room. We have seen it in paintings and films, framed as nostalgia. Yet when it happens in real life, it is anything but outdated. It is deeply human.

I was reminded of this when a longtime patient of mine chose hospice at home. I had cared for her for years—through routine visits, small worries, and larger battles. As her health declined, she made the decision to remain in her own home.

When I stepped into her bedroom, she was lying in her own bed, surrounded by family. The room felt sacred. Familiar photos on the walls. Soft light through the window. The hum of life continuing around her. When she saw me, tears welled in her eyes. She could hardly believe I had come. In that moment, no medication, no intervention, no order in the chart could equal the comfort of simply being present. The relationship had come full circle—from clinic exam room to bedside in her own home. There was something profoundly right about it.

Another patient—a gentleman with end-stage prostate cancer—made the decision not to pursue further treatment. He chose peace over prolongation. I visited him at home as well. He was thinner, quieter, but still unmistakably himself. He had stories—stories of youth, of work, of family, of a life well-lived. If time were unlimited, I would have stayed for hours just listening. Instead, I listened as long as I could, ensuring his symptoms were controlled, that he was comfortable, that nothing had been overlooked. I worked closely with the hospice nurse, making sure his final weeks were dignified, gentle, and free of unnecessary suffering. There is a privilege in caring for someone at the end of life in the space where their life actually happened.

And then there was her.

A woman in her 90s with stage IV breast cancer to the bone—given a grim prognosis, yet who went on to live nearly another decade. She had one clear wish: I want to die in my own home. She told me this more than once. It was not said casually. It was a declaration.

As she became bedridden, she could no longer come to clinic. For most patients, this is the point where placement in a skilled nursing facility becomes unavoidable. But she had a daughter—fiercely devoted—who chose to give her mother 24/7 care. Nursing-home-level care, delivered with love. Hydration maintained. Nutrition carefully managed. Hygiene impeccable. No pressure sores. No skin breakdown. No neglect. Only vigilance and sacrifice.

My nurse and I would stop by. We would check vitals, draw labs when needed and ship them to the lab, evaluate subtle changes. Sometimes the daughter would call: "She seems a bit different." We would assess for a UTI, an electrolyte imbalance—small, treatable issues that could otherwise spiral. The daughter was attentive. Competent. Exhausted, surely—but unwavering.

At one point, a vulnerable adult case was filed, alleging inadequate care. The county became involved—social workers, human services, the machinery of the system. There was talk of guardianship. Placement in a facility. Removing the daughter's authority.

They called me for my opinion.

I did not agree.

I had been there. I had seen the care. I had seen the devotion. There were no gaps. If anything, she was receiving more attentive care than many institutionalized patients ever do. Her wish had always been clear. She wanted to remain home.

The county offered home health. Hospice. Additional services. They were declined. Not out of denial—but out of clarity. The daughter was capable. The patient was lucid in her preference. Autonomy still mattered.

Eventually, the county backed off.

She continued to live at home for years. And when her time finally came, it came exactly where she had wanted it to—under her own roof, in her own bed, surrounded by what was familiar and loved. She died with dignity. Not because the system made it easy—it did not—but because her daughter made a sacrifice few can make, and because we, as her medical team, chose to support her wishes rather than override them.

These cases are rare. Most families cannot provide that level of care. Most circumstances force other outcomes. That is reality. But when it is possible—when love, commitment, and medical partnership align— there is something profoundly beautiful about it.

Losing a patient is never easy. Even when expected. Even when they are frail. Even when hospice is involved. Years of shared history do not disappear simply because death is anticipated. You remember their voice. Their expressions. Their stories. Their trust.

Home visits strip medicine down to its essence.

No fluorescent lights.

No rushing between rooms.

No institutional walls.

Just a physician, a patient, and the quiet acknowledgment that this chapter is closing.

It is not outdated.

It is medicine at its most human.

The First Death Certificate

When I first completed my medical residency and stepped into my role as an attending physician, I found myself practicing in a small rural town of about 13,000 people. It was a moment I had worked toward for years—finally independent, no longer supervised, entrusted fully with the care of my own patients. There was a deep sense of pride in that transition. I was seeing patients in clinic, rounding in the hospital, caring for residents in the nursing home, and being called upon across every setting where medicine touched lives. In a small town, the physician's role is not confined to walls or titles; you become woven into the fabric of the community.

Slowly, I began to build my own patient panel. These were no longer "assigned" patients or temporary encounters. These were my patients—people I would see repeatedly, sometimes weekly, sometimes monthly, often over years. Many carried complex medical histories, layered with chronic disease, frailty, and the realities of aging. Rural medicine, by its very nature, leans heavily into geriatrics. And for me, that felt natural.

I have always been passionate about rural health, but just as deeply about the care of the elderly. During my residency training, I had the privilege of working alongside some of the greatest geriatricians in the country. My institution housed a geriatrics fellowship program, and the culture of thoughtful, compassionate, patient-centered care left a lasting imprint on me. I learned that geriatrics is not simply about managing medications or diagnoses—it is about understanding goals, preserving dignity, and honoring lives rich with stories.

During residency, I was assigned two patients in the nursing home whom I followed continuously for three years until graduation. Over time, our relationship evolved beyond routine medical care. I learned their histories, their families, their fears, their humor. They came to recognize my voice and trust my presence. That experience bonded me to them and, unknowingly at the time, prepared me for the emotional realities of geriatric medicine. It taught me that continuity of care is not just a clinical advantage—it is a deeply human one.

So when I started my first attending job, caring for elderly patients felt like familiar territory. Many older adults established care with me, and over time, relationships grew. Trust was built slowly and organically. Conversations extended beyond labs and blood pressures. We spoke about spouses lost, children grown, regrets carried, and hopes still alive. In rural medicine, the boundary between physician and person often softens. You see your patients at the grocery store, at community events, sometimes in moments of joy, sometimes in moments of profound vulnerability.

Then comes the part of medicine no one can fully prepare you for.

One of my patients became seriously ill and was transferred to a large tertiary medical center. The illness progressed, and after thoughtful discussions with family and care teams, a decision was made to proceed with comfort measures only. The patient passed away shortly thereafter.

Not long after, I received an official document from the state: my first death certificate.

On paper, it was a form—clinical, administrative, procedural. In reality, it was a heavy and final acknowledgment of loss. I remember sitting with it, realizing that this was not an abstract patient or a distant case. This was someone I knew. Someone I had cared for, spoken with, laughed with. Someone who had trusted me.

That first death certificate had a profound impact on me. It affected me more than I ever expected. I felt a deep sadness that lingered for days. I questioned myself—not my clinical decisions, but my emotional readiness. Medical training prepares you to save lives, to diagnose, to treat. It does not fully prepare you for the quiet weight of finality.

With time, reality asserts itself. You learn that death is not a failure of medicine but an inevitability of life. The second and third death certificates arrive. Then more. Gradually, acceptance forms—not as indifference, but as understanding. Yet nothing quite compares to the first. It stays with you, etched into memory.

What many people may not realize is how deeply medical professionals bond with their patients. When you care for someone over many years, when you walk alongside them through illness, aging, and decline, they become more than a name on a chart. Sometimes, they begin to feel like family. Letting go is never easy.

But medicine is not about holding on at all costs. It is about doing what is best for the patient—even when that means stepping back, listening, and honoring their wishes. Sometimes the most compassionate care is not another procedure or intervention, but comfort. Hospice. Presence. Peace.

Caring for the elderly has taught me that dignity at the end of life is just as important as vitality at the beginning. It has taught me humility, empathy, and respect for the natural arc of human existence. And while death certificates may become more familiar with time, each one still represents a life lived, a story told, and a relationship that mattered.

That first certificate changed me. It made me a more reflective physician. A more human one. And it reaffirmed why I chose this path—to care, to connect, and to honor life in all its stages, even its final one.

The Luxury of Enough Time

There is a quiet tension in medicine that few outside the exam room ever see.

It lives in the space between what is right for a patient and what makes sense on a spreadsheet.

In rural clinics, especially those built on capitation, the math is simple. You are paid per patient, not per problem. From a business standpoint, it doesn't make sense to do too much in a single visit. One issue per appointment is tidy. Predictable. Profitable. A chronic disease follow-up today. The wart another day. The blood pressure now. The knee injection later.

Neat columns. Clean billing.

But patients are not columns.

They are people who drove 30 miles through snow to get there. People who took unpaid time off from a shift at the factory. People who found childcare, rearranged schedules, waited three weeks for an opening.

They walk in with hypertension—and a knee that has kept them up at night. Diabetes—and a stubborn wart their granddaughter keeps asking about. They don't think in CPT codes. They think in relief. In convenience. In hope that today, finally, everything can be handled.

And then comes the familiar phrase: "Let's schedule another appointment for that."

From the system's perspective, it is reasonable. From the patient's perspective, it can feel like rejection. As if their life must be divided into billable fragments.

I can put myself in their shoes. It is not fun to make multiple visits for different pieces of the same body. It is frustrating to finally see your doctor and be told that only one concern makes the cut today—even when both could be addressed safely in the same room, in the same hour.

The truth is uncomfortable: often, the system—not the provider—is to blame.

When payment models reward productivity, productivity becomes the north star. More visits. More encounters. More RVUs. The unspoken message is clear: see more, earn more. Efficiency is praised. Volume is applauded.

But something precious erodes in the process.

Time.

Time to listen without glancing at the clock. Time to freeze the wart after adjusting insulin. Time to inject the arthritic knee after reviewing the blood pressure log. Time to notice the subtle worry behind a patient's eyes.

In our rural clinic, we were fortunate. Volume and productivity were not the driving force. We were supported—truly supported—in doing everything reasonably possible for the patient in one visit.

We addressed chronic disease, skin and joint concerns, labs, screenings, vaccines. We performed minor procedures—skin biopsies, joint injections, cryotherapy for warts, removal of lesions. We tried to make the visit count.

Patients appreciated it in ways that numbers can't measure. Gratitude in their voices. Relief in their posture. "Thank you for taking care of all of it today." Those words carry weight.

I remain deeply thankful to our employer for never pressuring us to change our practices based on coding strategies or billing optimization. No subtle nudges to split visits unnecessarily. No reminders about missed revenue opportunities. Just trust—trust that we would do what was right.

Contrast that with productivity-based environments.

I have seen colleagues under those models. Talented, compassionate physicians—transformed by incentive structures. They were aggressive about filling schedules. When a patient no-showed or cancelled at the last minute, frustration surfaced immediately. That empty slot wasn't breathing room; it was lost income.

Meanwhile, a physician on a flat salary might see that same empty space differently. A chance to return patient calls. To refill medications thoughtfully. To review labs carefully. To catch up on documentation without cutting corners. To breathe.

The difference is subtle but profound.

One model asks, "How many did you see?"

The other asks, "How well did you care for them?"

I remember early in my career sitting across from the regional vice president. It was the beginning of my job, when everything still felt negotiable. She discussed compensation structures, productivity metrics, earning potential.

I told her plainly: I did not want a productivity model.

I wanted a flat salary.

I wanted the freedom to focus on my patients without calculating whether freezing a wart during a hypertension visit would disrupt financial efficiency. I did not want to favor quantity over quality. I did not want to feel a twinge of irritation at a no-show. I did not want the subtle pressure to shorten conversations that mattered.

I wanted to practice medicine the way it feels when you first decide to become a doctor.

Not hurried. Not transactional. Not fragmented.

Whole.

There is a misconception that doing more in one visit is reckless or unsafe. Certainly, care must be appropriate and manageable. But often, addressing two related concerns together is not dangerous—it is humane.

The rural patient does not experience their arthritis on Mondays and their diabetes on Thursdays. Their body is a single story unfolding in real time. They deserve a physician willing to read the whole chapter, not just the first paragraph.

Financial incentives will always exist. Systems will always calculate. That is reality.

But within those systems, there are choices.

Choices about how we structure compensation. Choices about what we reward. Choices about whether we measure value in encounters—or in trust.

When we align incentives with patient-centered care, something remarkable happens. The exam room feels less like a checkpoint and more like a sanctuary. Physicians feel less like production units and more like healers. Patients feel seen—not scheduled.

And perhaps that is the quiet revolution medicine needs.

Not louder productivity reports.

Just the courage to say: I choose quality. I choose wholeness. I choose the patient in front of me.

Every time.

What the Numbers Cannot See

Most healthcare systems are exceptionally good at measuring what is easily measurable. They can tell you, down to the decimal, how many patients you saw in a given month. They can calculate your RVUs with mathematical precision. They can generate colorful dashboards, productivity curves, and year-over-year comparisons. Numbers are clean. Numbers are tidy. Numbers are reportable.

But medicine—real medicine—rarely fits neatly into a spreadsheet.

The true work of a provider extends far beyond the exam room door and long after the clinic lights dim. Behind every appointment slot is a living, breathing panel of patients who depend on you in ways that cannot be captured by billing codes.

There is not a single day that goes by without the steady hum of messages, calls, refill requests, and urgent questions. Someone with a cold is immunosuppressed and anxious: "Should I hold my medication?" Another patient wakes with burning urination and pleads, "Can I just drop off a urine sample? I can't miss work." Someone else is experiencing dizziness from a new antihypertensive and wonders whether to cut the dose in half. A mother calls because her child's fever spiked at midnight. An elderly patient is confused about discharge instructions from a specialist. A pharmacy faxes a prior authorization. Another patient's insulin is about to run out because their insurance changed formularies without warning.

Then come the refill requests—dozens of them—each one requiring review: labs checked, renal function assessed, last visit noted, safety ensured. These are not clerical tasks; they are clinical decisions. Each click carries responsibility.

In many ways, this invisible work can be more time-consuming than the visits themselves. A fifteen-minute appointment may generate thirty minutes of follow-up. A hospital discharge triggers medication reconciliation, coordination with home health, and careful monitoring to prevent readmission. A simple lab abnormality leads to phone calls, counseling, repeat testing, documentation, and reassurance.

And then there is documentation—the ever-present companion. Notes waiting to be signed. Orders to co-sign. Messages to close. Charts that follow you home like unfinished conversations. Many physicians know the quiet ritual of opening the laptop after dinner, of catching up on charting while the rest of the house sleeps. Weekends become administrative recovery time. The cognitive load of medicine does not end when clinic ends.

Layered onto this is the labyrinth of insurance: prior authorizations, peer-to-peer reviews, formulary substitutions, denials that require appeals. Time spent explaining to a non-clinician why a patient truly needs the medication you prescribed. Time defending decisions that were made thoughtfully, compassionately, and appropriately.

None of this generates RVUs.

Yet all of it generates value.

This behind-the-scenes work—often invisible to the employer—is as important, if not more important, than face-to-face encounters. It prevents complications. It reduces hospitalizations. It builds trust. It strengthens continuity. It keeps patients safe. It is the glue that holds together the fragmented pieces of modern healthcare.

I was fortunate to work with a clinic director who understood this deeply. He came from a clinical background. He knew that the worth of a physician cannot be reduced to throughput. He understood that value is not only in volume.

We built a relationship rooted in mutual respect and trust. He managed operations; I managed the medical side as medical director. There was clarity in our roles and confidence in each other's judgment. He never hovered over providers demanding more patients per hour. He never reduced conversations to productivity metrics alone.

Even when pressure came from the "mothership"—the larger system focused on numbers—he advocated for us. He prepared reports not just of RVUs, but of impact. He highlighted leadership roles, teaching responsibilities, quality improvement initiatives, community outreach efforts, nursing home coverage, hospital work, committee participation, mentorship of new providers. He translated invisible labor into language the system could understand.

In many ways, he stood up for his physicians and providers. That kind of leadership is rare and refreshing. It creates psychological safety. It allows physicians to practice good medicine instead of fast medicine. It reminds providers that they are seen—not just counted.

I consider myself truly blessed that in every position I have held so far, I have worked with sensible, thoughtful directors. Leadership can either drain the joy from medicine or protect it. When leaders understand the full spectrum of a provider's contribution, the job becomes lighter. The work becomes sustainable. The mission feels shared.

Because at the end of the day, medicine is not a production line. It is a covenant. Patients entrust us with their fears, their vulnerabilities, their lives. The work we do—both visible and invisible—honors that trust.

And no metric can fully measure that.

Medicine in an Age of Metrics

There was a time when the only "rating" a physician received was a quiet nod from a recovering patient, a handshake from a grateful family, or the unspoken trust of a community. Today, that same physician may be distilled into a number—4.5 or 4.8—displayed beside a headshot like a boutique hotel on a travel website. The modern healthcare system calls this progress. And perhaps it is. But perhaps it is also something else.

Healthcare did not become consumer-driven by accident. Patients now comparison-shop, read reviews, schedule online, and expect transparency. In a world where restaurants, rides, and retail are rated in real time, medicine was unlikely to remain untouched. Healthcare systems argue, with some logic, that if they do not measure patient experience themselves, others will do it for them. Anonymous platforms already allow unverified commentary and emotional reactions to shape reputations. By creating structured satisfaction systems, institutions attempt to verify encounters, standardize feedback, and protect physicians from malicious or fabricated reviews. From an administrative standpoint, this is rational. Reputation influences patient volume. Patient volume sustains hospitals. In competitive and rural markets alike, perception can determine survival.

And yet, something shifts when the polished consultant stands before a room of physicians and explains—with elegant slides and corporate polish—that doctors are not so different from furniture salespeople. That we are in the business of customer satisfaction. The alarm rises quietly but unmistakably. A physician is not persuading someone to upgrade a sofa. We are not closing deals. We are entrusted with asymmetrical knowledge and fragile trust. Patients come anxious, vulnerable, and often afraid. They are not browsing; they are seeking counsel. The comparison fails not because service does not matter, but because the ethical framework is entirely different. A salesperson's duty is to close the transaction. A physician's duty is to tell the truth—even when it disappoints. Especially when it disappoints.

Is a physician with a 4.5-star rating worse than one with a 4.8? What do those three-tenths truly represent? Perhaps clearer explanations and warmer bedside presence. Perhaps more time spent listening. Or perhaps more antibiotics prescribed for viral infections, more imaging ordered "just in case," more agreement when evidence demanded restraint. A physician practicing strict evidence-based medicine may, by necessity, disappoint more often. Saying no is rarely satisfying in the moment. Declining a test read about online. Refusing an antibiotic for a viral cold. Advising against a medication that helped a neighbor. You explain carefully. You educate. You reason. And still, the patient may leave unsatisfied.

Could it be that the 4.5-star physician is more current with the literature, more disciplined with stewardship, more committed to long-term outcomes, while the 4.8-star physician is more accommodating? Or could it be the opposite—that dissatisfaction often reflects not principled refusal but poor communication? Perhaps many negative surveys are not about being told no, but about not feeling heard before the no was delivered. Satisfaction may reflect empathy as much as acquiescence. And here lies the tension: medicine exists at the intersection of biology and expectation. You can align physiology with evidence. You cannot always align desire with reality.

Should we say yes to every request? If patient satisfaction becomes the dominant metric, subtle incentives shift. The calculus changes—short-term harmony versus long-term stewardship, individual happiness versus population health. The danger is rarely dramatic corruption; it is incremental drift. One unnecessary antibiotic to avoid conflict. One imaging study to prevent a complaint. One prescription added to preserve a score. Multiply that by thousands of encounters, and culture quietly transforms.

Yet to dismiss patient satisfaction entirely would be equally shortsighted. Communication matters. Empathy matters. Feeling respected matters. A technically brilliant physician who dismisses concerns erodes trust, and without trust, adherence falters and outcomes suffer. Medicine is not merely the correct diagnosis; it is the relationship that allows the diagnosis to be accepted and the plan to be followed. In that sense, patient satisfaction measures something real and important. It captures the patient's lived experience of care, the human side of clinical practice that no lab value can quantify.

Healthcare systems, meanwhile, operate within economic realities. When one institution markets "five-star care," others inevitably follow. Trends become expectations. Administrators insist they are protecting physicians by centralizing ratings rather than leaving reputations to anonymous online platforms. They want verified feedback and institutional oversight. There is truth in that. But there is also branding. Public scorecards. Star icons beside credentials earned through years of sacrifice and training. Medicine has entered the marketplace of perception, whether we welcome it or not.

The deeper question is not about surveys. It is about identity. Is medicine a service industry? In part, yes. Is it a business? Unavoidably. Is it a calling grounded in fiduciary duty? Absolutely. The danger lies not in measuring patient experience, but in mistaking it for the whole story. Satisfaction measures how a patient feels. It does not measure diagnostic accuracy, complication rates, or adherence to evolving guidelines. A pleasant misdiagnosis can still be catastrophic. A firm, unpopular decision can still be lifesaving.

There are other ways to measure excellence: risk-adjusted outcomes, evidence-based practice patterns, complication rates, peer review, continuing education, case complexity, work ethic. These metrics are harder to condense into stars. Harder to display on a billboard. Harder to translate into marketing language. Stars are simple. Excellence rarely is.

Perhaps the answer is not to reject patient satisfaction nor to enthrone it. Perhaps it belongs as one instrument in a larger orchestra. A useful signal, but not the conductor. The physician's compass must remain oriented toward evidence, ethics, and patient welfare. Sometimes that compass points toward agreement. Sometimes it points toward principled refusal.

A 4.5-star physician may be practicing harder medicine. A 4.8-star physician may be practicing kinder communication. Either could be excellent. Either could be compromised. The real measure of a doctor is not fully captured in decimal points. It is found in the quiet moments after the visit ends, when the door closes and there is no audience, no survey, no applause—only the question: Did I act in this patient's best medical interest, even if it cost me half a star?

That is a metric no platform can quantify. And perhaps that is precisely why the conversation must continue.

Leadership Beyond the Bubble: Rethinking What Healthcare Leadership Should Look Like

Leadership in healthcare takes many forms. Over the years, I have experienced a wide spectrum of styles—some inspiring, some transactional, some disconnected from the clinical reality. Titles alone do not determine leadership. Background matters. Mindset matters more. But proximity to the front line matters most.

There are many recognized approaches to leadership: transformational leaders who cast vision and inspire; transactional leaders who focus on metrics and targets; servant leaders who prioritize the needs of staff and patients; collaborative and participatory leaders who share decision-making; authoritative leaders who provide direction and control; laissez-faire leaders who step back; dyad models that pair physician and administrator; and the simple but powerful practice of management by walking around. In healthcare, no single style fits every situation. Yet certain qualities consistently rise to the surface—partnership, visibility, humility, and a deep respect for the realities of patient care.

In medicine, leaders with a clinical background often hold an advantage. They understand the exam room. They understand the hospital floor at 2 a.m. They understand the weight of uncertainty and the quiet burden that does not show up in a spreadsheet. But administrators without medical training can also be highly effective—if they truly partner with their physician counterparts. The dyad works when both sides respect the other's expertise and compensate for one another's blind spots. It fails when one side pretends to understand what they have never lived.

I once worked with a clinic director whose entire worldview revolved around numbers—productivity metrics, percentages, dashboards. He had an MBA and could recite statistics with ease. But he had no understanding of what happens inside a clinic room with a patient. No appreciation for nuance, for silence, for grief, for complexity. Everything became throughput.

In contrast, I worked with another administrator who began as a physical therapist before transitioning into leadership. He understood the human side of medicine instinctively. Conversations about patient care did not require translation. You could speak about moral tension, about the gray zones, and he would simply nod—he got it. He protected his staff. He stood up to higher administration when necessary. He understood that medicine is not merely a business model; it is a human encounter. His success did not come from authority. It came from understanding.

A strong CEO brings vision, mission, and values. That is essential. But vision without partnership becomes isolation. The most effective executive I work with pairs vision with presence. She partners closely with clinical leaders and remains meaningfully engaged in the realities of frontline care. She understands that leadership is not sitting in an office receiving polished summaries and filtered reports—because the truth rarely travels upward unchanged. Instead, she creates space for direct conversation, for unvarnished feedback, and for hearing what is actually happening rather than what is convenient to report. She is also a clear and intentional practitioner of the dyad model, fostering true physician–administrator partnership rather than symbolic alignment. That structure has not only strengthened communication and accountability across the organization, it has made her leadership measurably more effective.

CEOs who remain in the background, attending a few meetings and receiving rosy reports, are often left in the dark. I would suggest they step out of the bubble. Present to the front line. Talk directly to nurses, physicians, receptionists. Make rounds with inpatient teams. Visit rural clinics. Sit down and ask simple questions: What is working? What is not? What is keeping you from doing your job well?

If you want the truth, you must seek it yourself. Do not rely solely on reports prepared by others.

Organizations frequently distribute employee satisfaction surveys that claim to be anonymous. Yet many employees do not trust them. I cannot count how many colleagues have admitted they filter their responses for fear of retaliation. When fear shapes feedback, honesty disappears. Perhaps the old-fashioned way still has merit—a simple comment box where staff can write concerns and drop them in. Not monitored by a camera, of course. Sarcasm aside, trust is fragile. It is earned when leaders prove that candor is safe.

Communication matters as well. Automated holiday emails—long, polished, wordy—are often deleted within seconds. No one reads them. They click delete. The message is buried under corporate phrasing. Instead of an automated or AI-generated message, write one line. Large. Bold. Personal: "Merry Christmas. I appreciate everything you do for our patients. I admire every one of you." Your own words. Authenticity carries more weight than eloquence.

In large healthcare systems, senior administrators can become so far removed from daily reality that their emails unintentionally reveal the distance. Sometimes the ignorance is so evident that employees' jaws drop. It is not always ill intention. Often it is insulation.

So what is a successful leader?

It is someone hands-on and visible. Humble. Approachable. Someone you can request a face-to-face meeting with and receive it without conditions. Someone in contact with frontline workers. Someone who does not rely solely on reports but seeks the truth personally. Someone available.

A successful leader knows their weaknesses. If they do not come from a medical background, they rely deeply on their medical counterparts rather than pretending to know it all. They protect their staff when necessary. They cannot be manipulated by the few who surround them with selective narratives. They use both data and intuition to make decisions. They can put themselves in the shoes of their employees without effort. They understand the emotional labor of medicine.

This may sound harsh. But reflection is necessary.

Healthcare is not a factory. It is not merely a balance sheet. It is a living system built on trust, responsibility, and human vulnerability. Leadership in such a system cannot be distant. It cannot be automated. It cannot be insulated.

It must walk the halls.

It must sit in the clinic room.

It must listen without defense.

And above all, it must remember that behind every metric is a patient, and behind every patient is a team that deserves to be seen, heard, and protected.

The Quiet Work Behind the Scenes: Where Medicine Meets the Margin

One of the quiet tensions in modern medicine is not the complexity of disease, nor even the emotional weight of difficult diagnoses.

It is the relationship between clinical judgment and insurance structure.

There are many insurance companies, each with its own formulary, its own processes, its own thresholds for approval. The lack of uniformity can be challenging. What is covered under one plan may require prior authorization under another. A medication that is first-line in one system may require step therapy in the next. The variability itself becomes part of the clinical landscape.

To be fair, some of their concerns are legitimate. Overutilization of imaging, unnecessary procedures, and indiscriminate prescribing are real issues in American healthcare. Resources are finite. Costs matter. Guardrails are necessary.

But guardrails should guide care—not obstruct it. Cost containment should never come at the expense of patient safety, clinical outcomes, or timely decision-making.

Prior authorization offers a clear example. A patient presents with abdominal pain. Based on history and examination, a CT abdomen is appropriate. In many cases, prior authorization is required before the scan can be obtained. The review process can be thoughtful and reasonable—but when it becomes prolonged in a time-sensitive situation, clinical momentum is lost.

If approval is delayed, the patient may ultimately be referred to the emergency department. Now the system pays not only for the imaging and labs, but also for the ER visit. A process designed to ensure appropriate utilization can inadvertently increase both cost and complexity.

Medication coverage presents similar nuances. Favoring generics over high-cost brand medications when efficacy is equivalent is responsible stewardship. But sometimes a low-cost generic is not covered, or the suggested alternatives are not therapeutically comparable. When substitutions are clinically mismatched, delay and instability can follow.

The administrative layer also adds time. The initial visit includes history, examination, assessment, documentation, and treatment planning. When additional letters of medical necessity or peer-to-peer discussions are required, it extends the work well beyond the patient encounter. The intention is oversight; the impact is often increased administrative burden.

Hospital admission determinations can be particularly complex.

An 18-year-old woman arrives with flank pain, vomiting, a fever of 104°F, heart rate 115, and borderline blood pressures. CRP greater than 400. WBC 24,000. Markedly elevated procalcitonin. CT abdomen and pelvis with IV contrast shows unilateral pyelonephritis with possible perinephric abscess.

Clinically, she is septic.

In a larger hospital, she might have been admitted to an ICU. In our small rural facility without an ICU, she was admitted to the medical floor for IV antibiotics, IV fluids, close monitoring, and cultures. Within forty-eight hours, her fever subsided, her pain improved, and urine culture data guided therapy. She was discharged on appropriate oral antibiotics. Her blood cultures remained negative.

Weeks later, a letter arrived.

Denied.

"Patient did not warrant inpatient admission."

A peer-to-peer discussion was offered. The conversation centered on the negative blood cultures. The implication was that without bacteremia, the admission was unnecessary.

But clinical decisions are made prospectively, based on presentation—not retrospectively, based on outcomes. Sepsis does not require bacteremia. Stability on day three does not negate instability on day one. We do not have the privilege of hindsight at the bedside.

The denial stood. An appeal was submitted.

Two years later, there has been no response.

These situations are not uncommon. An MRI deferred until six weeks of therapy have elapsed, even when function is severely limited. A continuous glucose monitor approved only after another hypoglycemic episode. An anticoagulant changed repeatedly as formularies shift. An elderly patient destabilized because a familiar inhaler is no longer preferred.

Each denial requires time. Each appeal demands explanation. Each phone call competes with direct patient care.

None of this makes insurers adversaries. Their role in managing population-level costs and preventing misuse is important. Healthcare requires stewardship. Accountability matters.

But the system functions best when cost-awareness and clinical judgment operate in alignment rather than tension. Oversight should refine care—not delay it. Stewardship should enhance outcomes—not risk them.

At the center of all of this is the patient.

The young woman with a 104-degree fever. The diabetic trying to steady unpredictable blood sugars. The patient in pain waiting for imaging. They do not see the administrative exchanges. They experience only whether care arrives in time.

The shared goal—physicians and insurers alike—should be simple: appropriate care, delivered at the right time, without compromising safety or sustainability.

Medicine is practiced in moments. Policy is written in patterns. The challenge is ensuring that when those two meet, the patient remains the priority.

The Promise Behind the Premium

Health insurance is one of those things almost everyone has… and almost no one fully understands.

You see it when the bill comes.

You feel it when a claim is denied.

You hear about it when premiums go up.

But the machinery behind it? That is mostly invisible.

At its heart, insurance is simple. It is a promise. We all put money into a shared pot so that when one of us gets sick, the cost does not destroy a family. It is community at scale.

Over time, that simple promise became a very complex system.

Medicare was created so our elders would not grow old and sick without care. Before it existed, many seniors simply went without treatment. Today, it covers hospital stays, clinic visits, medications — though not everything. There are still deductibles and copays, which is why many people buy supplemental plans.

As we live longer — and we are living much longer — care becomes more complicated and more expensive. Joint replacements. Cancer treatments. Heart procedures. Dialysis. Miracles of modern medicine that were once unimaginable. Medicare carries much of that weight. It is essential. Hard to imagine life without it. Yet as the population ages, the financial pressure grows. More beneficiaries. Fewer workers supporting the system. The math becomes tight.

Medicaid exists for those with limited income — children, pregnant mothers, people with disabilities, the elderly in nursing homes. It is a quiet lifeline. Many people do not realize that Medicaid pays for a large share of long-term nursing home care in America. Without it, many families would face impossible choices.

It too strains under rising costs. Healthcare does not get cheaper. Technology advances. Expectations rise. Needs increase.

Then there is private insurance, often tied to employment. Hundreds of companies. Different rules. Different networks. Different formularies. One plan covers a medication easily; another requires layers of approval. One hospital is "in network." Another is not.

To the patient, it can feel random.

To the clinic, it means phone calls, forms, prior authorizations, appeals.

To employers, it means yearly negotiations and rising premiums.

We spend about 17–18% of our entire economy on healthcare — more per person than almost any other country. A meaningful portion of that spending goes to administration: billing systems, claims processing, compliance, paperwork. Money that moves through offices instead of exam rooms.

There are other invisible forces too. Fear of lawsuits can nudge doctors toward extra tests. Payment models sometimes reward doing more rather than doing better. Prices for the same service can vary wildly depending on contracts few people ever see.

From the outside, it looks chaotic.

From the inside, it feels layered — decades of policy decisions stacked on top of one another, rarely erased, only added to.

And here is the part most people never hear: almost no one fully understands all of it. Not patients. Not doctors. Not administrators. Not even policymakers. Each person sees one corner of the maze.

The debates you hear — raising eligibility ages, expanding coverage, reducing fraud, moving toward value-based care, simplifying administration — are attempts to answer one hard question:

How do we care for everyone, fairly and sustainably, in a world where medicine can do more than ever before — but never for free?

Insurance is not just contracts and premiums.

It is our collective decision that illness should not mean ruin.

That aging should not mean abandonment.

That vulnerability should not mean isolation.

The structure may need reshaping. The inefficiencies should be addressed. Waste and fraud should be reduced. Incentives can be improved. But underneath the bureaucracy and confusion is something profoundly human:

A shared agreement that when one of us falls, the rest help carry the weight.

If you have ever felt confused by the system, you are not behind. You are not uninformed. You are standing in front of one of the most complex financial and social structures ever built.

And you are not alone in trying to make sense of it.

Leaving the Keys on the Counter

There was a time when solo practice was the backbone of American medicine. A physician hung a shingle, opened the doors, and cared for a community for decades. Decisions were personal. Autonomy was absolute. Medicine felt simple.

But medicine is no longer simple.

As healthcare has grown more complex—with evolving regulations, billing requirements, coding intricacies, insurance negotiations, quality metrics, and compliance mandates—the number of solo practitioners has steadily declined. In some states, regulatory structure and market dynamics still allow solo practices to survive more easily than others, but the trend is undeniable: independent, one-physician clinics are becoming rare.

When I moved to a town of 4,500 people to begin my practice, I joined a health system. At the time, there were two physicians in town who maintained solo practices. They were content. They were their own bosses. No administrator dictated productivity targets. No system policies shaped their workflow. They practiced medicine on their own terms.

But independence comes at a cost.

Behind the exam room door lies an entire business operation—billing, coding, collections, payer negotiations, staffing, payroll, compliance, equipment maintenance, IT infrastructure, regulatory audits. Recruiting and retaining qualified staff is increasingly difficult. Competing with large health systems that offer comprehensive retirement plans, health insurance, disability coverage, and other benefits is nearly impossible for a small clinic. Every expense falls directly on the physician-owner.

Neither of those practices had implemented an electronic medical record system—likely due to cost and perhaps comfort with familiarity. Walking into their clinics felt like stepping back into 1990. Paper charts.

Fax machines humming. A rhythm of medicine that felt personal and unhurried. They had loyal patients who trusted them deeply, and for years, that model worked.

Retirement, however, presents another layer of complexity for the solo physician. When you own the practice, closing the door is not simple. Records must be maintained for years. Phone lines and fax machines must remain active. Patients need assistance transitioning to new providers. What should be a peaceful chapter of life can instead become administratively burdensome.

One of those physicians approached retirement and made a wise decision: he sold his practice to a larger health system. He merged, transitioned his patients into an established network, and gradually tapered down his clinical workload over several years before fully retiring. His patients found continuity. He left medicine with the reassurance that the people he had cared for would continue to be cared for. That, perhaps, is the greatest comfort a physician can have at the end of a career.

As for me, I cannot imagine running my own practice.

I want to walk into a clinic, see patients, diagnose, treat, comfort, and heal. I want to focus on medicine—the art and science I trained for and remain passionate about. I do not want to negotiate insurance contracts, manage payroll, oversee laboratory operations, handle equipment repairs, recruit staff, or troubleshoot IT failures. I respect those who thrive in that dual role of physician and entrepreneur, but I know myself well enough to understand where my strengths and passions lie.

For me, practicing within a system allows clarity of purpose. I can dedicate my energy to patient care, leadership, and improving clinical quality—without being consumed by the operational machinery that keeps a clinic running.

Solo practice may embody autonomy and nostalgia. System-based practice may sacrifice some independence. But ultimately, each model serves a different personality and philosophy of medicine.

In the end, what matters most is not the structure—it is that our patients are cared for, our communities are served, and we practice in a way that allows us to sustain both our calling and ourselves.

Between Allegiance and Oath

When I finished my training in a 500-bed hospital, I thought I had seen politics at its finest—committee meetings layered over committee meetings, quiet alliances in fluorescent hallways, power that flowed through titles and tenure. When I chose rural medicine, I believed I was stepping away from all of that. I imagined something simpler. Closer to patients. Farther from politics.

I was wrong.

The town was small, but its medical ecosystem was anything but simple. Four clinics and one hospital served a wide rural catchment area. Two clinics were run by solo physicians—independent, self-made, operating on instinct, resilience, and thin margins. The other two belonged to healthcare systems headquartered in a nearby city. Each brought its own culture, strengths, and resources into our shared community.

The hospital was city-owned and independent but managed by one of those systems. The other system also maintained a strong presence in town. The dynamics were rarely dramatic, but they were real—subtle differences in culture, communication styles, and operational priorities. One system's clinic focused heavily on obstetrics, caring for mothers and newborns, filling the halls with the first cries of life. The other leaned into geriatrics, walking patients through the later chapters of theirs. Different niches. Both necessary. Both serving the same community.

There has always been more than enough work for everyone. The catchment area is broad, the needs endless. And while affiliations naturally shape perspectives, I have come to appreciate how much shared purpose exists beneath those differences. Pride in one's organization is not a flaw; it often reflects commitment to standards and values. The key is ensuring that pride strengthens care rather than narrows collaboration.

On paper, everyone has equal hospital privileges. Equal participation. Equal rights. In practice, balancing local relationships with broader organizational structures requires awareness and maturity from all of us. The solo physicians safeguard their autonomy while contributing deeply to the hospital's mission. The system-employed physicians navigate both community expectations and organizational responsibilities. Each group carries unique pressures. Each plays an essential role.

Over time, I came to see that loyalty—to a system, to a clinic, to a way of practicing—has boundaries. Loyalty can foster unity, consistency, and shared standards. But it must always remain secondary to the patient in front of us. When we remember that, collaboration becomes far easier.

And when a patient decompensates in the ER, when a labor turns complicated, when a stroke alert sounds at 2 a.m., distinctions disappear. We trust each other's clinical judgment. We show up. We do the work. In those moments, what defines us is not affiliation but professionalism. Patient care cuts through everything else.

Rural medicine does not eliminate politics; it compresses them. In larger centers, politics are diluted across layers of administration. In a small town, everything is personal. You see one another at the grocery store. Your children attend the same schools. Board decisions echo through community conversations. Proximity magnifies dynamics—but it also creates opportunity for deeper trust.

Leadership in this setting is less about authority and more about stewardship. Titles matter far less than credibility. Relationships outlast contracts. Neutrality builds confidence. Transparency prevents misunderstanding. Ego—if allowed to dominate—becomes costly in ways that small communities feel quickly.

It is entirely possible to operate within different systems and still function as one medical community. That requires intentional professionalism. It means choosing language carefully. It means assuming good intent. It means consistently redirecting attention to the shared mission we all serve.

I arrived in rural medicine believing I had left politics behind. Instead, I found a more intimate version of it—one that demands nuance, humility, and emotional intelligence. It has challenged me more than I expected.

We may not all wear the same badge. But we serve the same town. In a community large enough for every clinic to thrive, the real work of rural leadership is not minimizing differences—it is ensuring they never overshadow care.

In the end, the patient remains the only flag worth defending.

On the Receiving End of Care

On Mondays, I go to work and step into my other life—the hospital corridors, the overhead pages, the steady rhythm of decisions that carry weight. Back home, my wife runs a different kind of hospital.

She works full time. She gets our 12- and 4-year-old boys up, dressed, fed, and delivered to school. She weaves through drop-offs and pick-ups, after-school practices and school events, grocery runs wedged between carpools, dinner on the table, homework supervised, laundry folded, fevers soothed. Some weeks, when I really think about it, I'm not sure I work harder than she does. What she does is essential work—unpaid overtime in the currency of love and responsibility.

It was the height of flu season when she called.

Our 12-year-old had woken up with fever, chills, body aches, and a sore throat. He stayed home from school. Influenza was everywhere. Strep was making its rounds too. As a physician, I know sometimes information is power. Strep is treatable. Certain strains of group A strep, if left untreated, can lead to rheumatic fever. Treatment shortens illness and limits spread. And if we knew what he had, we'd know what to expect if the rest of us—my wife, our 4-year-old—started showing symptoms.

Clarity matters.

I told her to take him to the closest urgent care and request influenza and strep testing. Simple swabs. Quick answers.

She loaded both boys into the car.

They sat.

Forty-five minutes later, my phone rang again. My wife's voice was tight. Our son had a high fever now. He was shivering, aching, head pounding. He couldn't sit upright in that plastic chair any longer. He just wanted to lie down. If you've ever had influenza, you know that feeling—the way your bones seem to hum with pain, the way gravity feels heavier than usual.

The urgent care isn't my own clinic or hospital, but it's one where I pick up shifts from time to time. I know many of the providers. I checked the schedule on my phone and called the clinician on shift.

"It's very busy," she said.

I understood. I live that reality. Still, I asked if she could place the orders so a nurse could collect the swabs. Straightforward. Efficient.

She paused. "The protocol requires everyone has to be seen first."

Another thirty minutes passed.

My wife called again. Still in the lobby. Not roomed. Our son pale and shivering, slumped against her shoulder. Our four-year-old restless beside them.

In that moment, I wasn't a physician with connections. I was a father, listening to the fatigue in my wife's voice and picturing my son's glassy eyes.

I told them to go home.

He took ibuprofen and crawled into bed. Curtains drawn. The house quiet except for the occasional cough. I called a physician friend, explained the situation. She didn't hesitate. "Of course," she said. Minutes later, she texted: Orders are in.

That afternoon, my wife returned to urgent care. With orders already placed, there was no debate. They collected the swabs.

The results came back later that day.

Influenza positive.

Strep negative.

There was relief in that clarity. No antibiotics needed. No looming worry about untreated strep. Just influenza—the kind that flattens you for days and humbles even the strongest twelve-year-old.

As the week unfolded, it moved through our house just as we suspected it would. A scratchy throat here. A low-grade fever there. The four-year-old curled up under a blanket that never stays on him long. My wife pushing through until she couldn't. But because we had that initial answer, there was less uncertainty. No repeat visits. No guessing. We managed it with hydration, rest, fever reducers, quiet rooms, patience. Soup simmering on the stove. Water bottles refilled. Thermometers beeping in the dark.

Information didn't cure the flu.

But it steadied us.

As physicians, we move through the healthcare system with fluency. We know the terminology. We know who to call. We understand workflows and policies. Even then, we encounter friction. We wait. We're redirected. We feel the quiet frustration of sitting in a lobby while a sick child shivers beside us.

If it feels that way for us—connected, medically literate, comfortable advocating—what does it feel like for the single parent who doesn't know which clinic to choose? For the elderly patient who can't drive across town? For the family missing hourly wages just to sit in that same chair?

We talk about policies, about standardization, about throughput. Necessary things. But from the other side of the front desk, those same systems can feel rigid. Impersonal.

Being on the receiving end is clarifying.

It exposes the small kinks in the machine—the required visit that makes sense on paper but not when your child has a 103-degree fever. It shows you where small changes could make a meaningful difference—

standing nurse-driven protocols during peak flu season, clearer communication, flexibility when appropriate.

More than anything, it softens you.

You pause longer.

You explain more clearly.

You look for ways to remove one unnecessary barrier.

Because when a parent calls twice asking how much longer it will be, they're not being difficult. They're watching their child suffer. When someone asks, "Do we really need another visit?" they may be calculating childcare, gas money, exhaustion.

Walking through the system as a father—not as a physician—didn't make me cynical. It made me attentive.

Every patient in that waiting room is someone's twelve-year-old. Someone's four-year-old. Someone's exhausted spouse.

Sometimes the greatest education in medicine doesn't happen in residency or conferences.

It happens in a plastic chair, in a crowded lobby, while your child leans against you and whispers, "Dad, can we go home?"

When the World Stood Still and Medicine Carried On

A new strain of coronavirus shook the world.

Our immune systems had never seen it before. There was no memory, no rehearsal, no quiet antibody waiting in reserve. The body struggled to recognize the threat. And so did we.

Hospitals filled with a mysterious pneumonia. Some patients with no significant risk factors deteriorated with stunning speed—placed on ventilators they would never leave. Others at the extremes of age, burdened with every known comorbidity, somehow survived. There was no reliable pattern. No predictable course. Medicine, so often guided by probability, was forced into humility.

We stopped elective surgeries. Routine care was suspended. Wellness exams, cancer screenings, chronic disease follow-ups for hypertension and diabetes, childhood vaccinations—all deferred. Clinics that once focused on prevention became centers of containment. Hallways turned into surge units. Resources were drained.

And then came the shortages.

Medications. Supplies. Staff.

PPE became precious.

We reused masks meant for a single shift for an entire week. N95s were scarce, guarded, recycled for days upon days. Straps frayed. Paper bags with handwritten names lined shelves. We made do because there was no alternative.

Nurses close to retirement left the workforce. Healthcare workers with underlying conditions stepped away to protect themselves. Some became sick. We lost colleagues. Burnout was not theoretical—it was visible in exhausted eyes above fogged goggles. Healthcare careers grew less attractive; training pipelines slowed; college outputs dropped. The workforce thinned while the need intensified.

We separated patients with respiratory symptoms from everyone else. You could not mix suspected COVID with children there for routine care in the same waiting room. We restructured clinics overnight. Outdoor testing sites appeared in parking lots. We pivoted to phone and video visits for respiratory complaints. Medicine—so grounded in human touch—became distant and digital.

It was a terrifying time.

Visitors were restricted. Some patients died without a loved one at the bedside to hold their hand. Families said goodbye through screens. In nursing homes, relatives stood outside windows, waving through glass at parents and grandparents they could not embrace. The most vulnerable—elderly residents, disabled patients in group homes, institutionalized individuals—bore the heaviest burden.

Inside hospital walls, providers waited for evidence-based treatment to emerge. Viral illnesses rarely yield quick cures. We watched data unfold in real time. Caution prevailed; no one wanted to cause harm in the rush to help. We waited for the green light before giving dexamethasone. Science moved deliberately, even as suffering moved quickly. There was frustration, uncertainty, restraint.

Meanwhile, another crisis grew quietly.

Patients stayed home.

Fear of contracting COVID kept them from clinics and emergency rooms. Hypertension went unchecked. Diabetes follow-ups were postponed. Cancer screenings were delayed. Preventive care stalled. Vaccinations were missed. By the time the acute wave subsided, some returned with advanced disease—complications that might have been prevented. This invisible damage may have been the most devastating of all.

Beyond medicine, society itself changed.

People could not travel. Could not gather. Could not socialize. Isolation strained mental health. Depression and anxiety deepened. Financial pressures mounted. Children learned through screens. Milestones passed quietly. Rituals of grief and celebration were altered. The fabric of society stretched thin—exposing both fragility and resilience.

Healthcare systems bent under relentless pressure. Supply chains proved fragile. Staffing models were strained. The trauma was not confined to ICUs—it seeped into every department, every clinic, every long-term care facility.

It was not simply a pandemic.

It was a tragedy.

It left scars in the minds of patients, in the hearts of their loved ones, in the spirits of providers, and in the structure of the entire healthcare system. It was post-traumatic stress experienced in real time—without pause, without distance, without the chance to process before the next wave arrived. We lived it as it unfolded. We carried it home after every shift.

Over time, the virus lost its overwhelming dominance—not because it vanished, but because humanity adapted. Through repeated exposure and the gradual development of herd immunity, its force diminished. It no longer silenced entire cities or overwhelmed hospitals in the same way. It joined the long list of respiratory viruses that circulate among us.

But we are not the same.

The workforce remains thinner. Burnout lingers. Trust must be rebuilt. Patients continue to catch up on delayed care. Mental health consequences persist. Structural weaknesses exposed during the crisis cannot be unseen.

History will document infection rates and mortality curves.

Those who lived it will remember something else:

The silence of restricted hospital rooms.

The hum of ventilators.

The ache behind reused masks.

The winter wind at outdoor testing sites.

The wave through nursing home windows.

The courage of staff who showed up anyway.

For a time, the world held its breath.

And in that suspended moment, medicine carried on—wounded, weary, creative, cautious, grieving, resilient.

A tragedy that scarred us.

A trauma shared in real time.

A chapter that reshaped healthcare, altered society, and reminded us how fragile—and how enduring—we truly are.

Beyond the Shift: The Human Cost of the Nursing Shortage

There are certain fractures in healthcare that do not make headlines the way pandemics do. They don't arrive overnight. They don't announce themselves with sirens.

They unfold quietly.

One shift short. One resignation email. One exhausted nurse who says, "I can't do this anymore."

And then another.

Post-COVID, one of the most persistent and destabilizing realities we've faced is the nursing shortage. Not a temporary dip. Not a seasonal fluctuation. A structural strain that continues to ripple through every corridor of every hospital.

You cannot run a hospital without nurses.

Not for an hour. Not for a shift. Not safely.

Physicians diagnose. Surgeons operate. Administrators strategize. But nurses are the constant presence—the eyes at the bedside at 2:17 a.m., the hands adjusting drips, the first to notice a subtle change in mentation, the ones who hear the fear in a patient's voice before it escalates into crisis.

When COVID struck, the strain was immediate. Nurses nearing retirement stepped away. Some left for safety. Some left from exhaustion. Others discovered different career paths or remote options and chose not to return. At the same time, nursing school enrollment dipped. The profession, at that moment, did not look inviting. It looked dangerous. It looked relentless. It looked unforgiving.

And the pipeline narrowed.

Hospitals began competing—not subtly, but aggressively. Sign-on bonuses grew. Hourly wages climbed. Incentives multiplied. Systems began recruiting from one another, unintentionally draining neighboring facilities to stabilize their own. What began as survival evolved into a bidding war.

Then the traveling nurse model exploded.

Staffing agencies negotiated premium contracts. Higher base pay. Housing stipends. Tax-advantaged allowances. Short-term commitments with long-term financial upside. For many nurses, it was an opportunity—financial freedom, flexibility, mobility.

For hospitals, it was both solution and gamble.

You rarely knew exactly who would walk through the door for that 13-week contract. Even when the nurse was excellent—and many were—the adjustment period was real. New electronic health record. New medication dispensing systems. New protocols. New culture. Every hospital has its own rhythm, its own unwritten rules. It takes time to practice at the top of your license in a new environment.

Time is a luxury we often didn't have.

Permanent staff felt the strain. They trained travelers while carrying their own assignments. Travelers carried heavy loads without the institutional memory that long-term staff possess. Burnout became a shared language.

And as nursing wages climbed—driven by market forces and mobility—physician and provider compensation largely stagnated. In some systems, it decreased.

At first glance, that disparity seems like it should trigger parallel mobility among physicians.

But it rarely does.

Changing jobs as a nurse can mean updating a resume and accepting a new contract within weeks. Changing jobs as a physician is an entirely different calculus.

Credentialing alone can take months—sometimes longer. Endless forms. Hospital committees. Payer enrollment. DEA registration updates. Privileging reviews. Background checks. If moving across state lines, add new licensure. State medical boards are not known for speed or simplicity.

Then there's malpractice coverage—claims-made versus occurrence, tail coverage negotiations. Disability insurance portability. Life insurance underwriting. Retirement account rollovers. Health insurance transitions. Non-compete clauses. Restrictive covenants.

None of it is simple.

And then there is the part that matters most—the human side.

By the time a physician is established in a community, they are not just employed. They are embedded.

You have a patient panel built over years. People who waited months to get in to see you. Families who refer their relatives because they trust your judgment. You know their histories without opening the chart. You remember who lost a spouse last winter. Whose child is applying to college. Who minimizes symptoms. Who catastrophizes.

If you are a PCP, walking away from that panel is not a financial decision. It is emotional. It feels, in some ways, like abandonment.

Within your organization, you are no longer "the new doctor." You are the steady one. The reliable one. The one nurses call when something feels off. The one administrators ask to weigh in on difficult decisions. The one colleagues trust in a code.

Move systems, and you start again.

New EHR. New politics. New culture. New leadership dynamics. New credibility to earn. You go from being deeply rooted to being a newcomer—proving yourself all over again.

For many physicians, that reset is heavier than any signing bonus is worth.

There are other anchors too.

Children settled in schools. Spouses with established careers. Aging parents nearby. Deep community ties. Leadership roles. Committee work. The quiet pride of belonging.

Money alone rarely dislodges that.

Meanwhile, hospitals continue to wrestle with staffing grids and coverage models. At the facilities I'm affiliated with, we regularly rely on traveling nurses to protect our core staff from burnout. It's a balancing act—stabilize the present without eroding the future.

We've explored creative solutions. International nurse recruitment. Sponsorship pathways. Long-term pipeline building. But immigration processes are slow, layered, and complex. Even with motivation, the timeline stretches into years.

So we adapt.

We cross-train. We flex schedules. We stretch budgets. We support the nurses who remain because without them, the system collapses.

And here's what often gets lost in the economic analysis:

Nurses are not interchangeable labor units.

They are culture carriers.

A seasoned nurse knows which physician prefers a direct page and which prefers a secure message. They anticipate needs before they are verbalized. They protect patients from system inefficiencies. They mentor younger staff. They anchor morale on difficult nights.

When shortages disrupt that continuity, something intangible erodes. The hospital still functions. The doors remain open. But the texture changes.

The stability feels thinner.

I do see a sliver of hope.

Interest in nursing appears to be rising again among younger generations. The profession is regaining visibility—not just as sacrifice, but as skill. As leadership. As impact. Educational programs are stabilizing. Applications are improving.

But pipelines take time.

A student entering nursing school today will not ease staffing pressures tomorrow. Clinical training. Licensure. Orientation. Experience. Competence grows in layers.

We are still in the middle of the lag.

What COVID revealed—brutally and without warning—is that healthcare is only as strong as the people willing to stand at the bedside. Titles matter less than presence. Infrastructure matters less than hands.

You cannot automate compassion. You cannot outsource vigilance. You cannot replace experience with policy.

The nursing shortage is not just a workforce issue. It is a relational issue. A sustainability issue. A reminder that healthcare is human at its core.

As physicians, we often speak about burnout in our own ranks—and rightly so. But we practice alongside colleagues who absorbed extraordinary trauma, loss, and pressure, often without the authority or autonomy that physicians hold.

They stayed. Or they left when they could no longer stay. Both decisions deserve respect.

If there is one lesson in all of this, it is this:

Healthcare does not function because of buildings.

It does not function because of reimbursement models.

It does not function because of strategy decks.

It functions because people show up.

And when fewer people are willing—or able—to show up, we feel it everywhere.

The path forward will not be quick. It will require pipeline investment, educational support, regulatory flexibility, cultural repair, and sustained leadership. It will require physicians and administrators to advocate not just for margins, but for meaning.

Because long after incentives fade and contracts expire, what remains are the relationships—the nurses who stand beside us in codes, the teams that weather difficult winters together, the shared glances across a crowded unit that say, "We've got this."

Staffing shortages test systems.

But they also reveal what holds them together.

And in every hospital I've walked through, even in the leanest seasons, what holds it together is still the same:

People who care enough to stay.

The Anatomy of Suffering in an Age of Fear

They say pain is a blessing.

Without it, we would not know when something inside us is breaking, bleeding, swelling, compressing, failing. Pain is the body's alarm system—ancient, protective, unsentimental. It startles us awake. It pulls our hand from the flame. It drives us toward help before damage becomes death.

In that sense, pain keeps us alive.

And yet, when pain becomes intense, unrelenting, and untreated, it transforms. The messenger becomes the tormentor. What was once protective becomes punishing.

Anyone who has endured severe physical pain—a fracture, a kidney stone, pancreatitis, postoperative agony—knows it is never just a sensation. It invades the mind. It corrodes dignity. It steals sleep, appetite, patience, hope. It narrows the world until all that remains is a single, merciless point of suffering.

So the question lingers, uncomfortable and persistent: How well do we treat pain in the hospital?

There was a time when pain was elevated—almost ceremonially—to the status of a vital sign. Alongside heart rate, blood pressure, respiratory rate, and temperature, pain was to be measured, documented, respected.

"On a scale of zero to ten…"

We asked. We charted. We tried.

But in the long shadow of the opioid epidemic—after the overdoses, the funerals, the headlines, the scrutiny—pain quietly lost its footing. Not officially. Not in policy manuals. But perceptibly. We still record it. We just do not always respond to it with the urgency we once promised.

Fear entered the room. And fear, unlike pain, is rarely charted.

Modern hospital pain control is structured, deliberate, algorithmic. Acetaminophen for mild pain. Oral opioids for moderate pain. Intravenous medication for severe breakthrough pain. PRN—as needed.

On paper, it is thoughtful. Balanced. Safe. A careful choreography designed to avoid excess while offering relief. Non-opioids are scheduled; opioids are held in reserve, guarded keys behind digital locks. It looks responsible.

And often, it is.

But the PRN system rests on something fragile. The patient must speak. The nurse must hear. The assessment must become action. The medication must be given. The cycle must repeat. Each step depends on attention, on trust, on judgment. When even one link weakens—a doubt, a delay, a distraction—pain goes untreated.

By morning rounds, the chart may show pain scores of seven, eight, nine, even ten. And the medication record may show nothing but acetaminophen.

The numbers tell one story. The patient's eyes tell another.

Pain has no laboratory value. No imaging study quantifies suffering. There is no biomarker for anguish. It is entirely subjective, and because it is subjective, it is vulnerable.

We are all human—physicians, nurses, care teams. We bring our histories with us. Some have watched addiction unravel a family. Some have seen respiratory depression steal a breath too many. Some carry memories of harm that make their hands cautious. Some believe patients exaggerate. Some unconsciously measure another's tolerance against their own. Some equate stoicism with legitimacy and visible distress with dramatization.

These biases do not announce themselves. They whisper. They show up as hesitation. A pause before clicking "administer." A preference for oral medication when intravenous might bring faster relief. A quiet hope that the pain will simply pass.

But pain does not care about our fears. It only cares that it is felt.

I remember an elderly gentleman who fell. Weeks later, after multiple emergency visits and clinic appointments, imaging showed what appeared to be a compression fracture. Once independent—driving, caring for family—he was now bedbound.

Because of pain.

When I admitted him for pain control, skepticism hovered in the background. Subtle, but present. Was this disproportionate? Was this low tolerance? Was something else at play?

One morning I reviewed his chart. Pain scores overnight: seven to ten. Medications administered: acetaminophen. His PRN opioids had not been given.

So we scheduled his oral medication. We spoke openly during rounds. We involved the team. And we obtained an MRI.

It was not a simple compression fracture. It was a burst fracture, potentially unstable.

He was transferred. He underwent kyphoplasty. He was discharged to rehabilitation. Weeks later, I heard he was more mobile, his pain improving, his independence slowly returning.

His suffering had not been exaggeration. It had been pathology. Pain had been telling the truth long before the imaging confirmed it.

Some conditions announce themselves with authority—acute fractures, pancreatitis, renal colic, postoperative incisions. Their legitimacy is rarely questioned. Others are quieter—cancer-associated pain, compression fractures, pelvic injuries. They may not look dramatic. They may not command the same urgency.

But they can devastate just as completely.

Pain does not always correlate with the drama of imaging. It does not follow our expectations. It does not obey our internal scale of what should hurt "that much." Sometimes the worst pain is the one we underestimate.

We are afraid—of respiratory depression, of sedation, of delirium, of addiction, of scrutiny, of judgment. These fears are not irrational. They are born of real tragedies and real harm.

But undertreated pain carries its own consequences. Immobility. Atelectasis. Delirium. Depression. Prolonged hospitalization. Loss of function. Loss of trust.

Pain control is not merely about comfort. It is about physiology. It is about recovery. It is about whether a patient can breathe deeply enough to avoid pneumonia, move enough to prevent a clot, rest enough to heal.

And it is about something even more fundamental.

Humanity.

In this age of fear, we have become careful—perhaps necessarily so. But careful must not become indifferent. Cautious must not become dismissive.

Pain is still the body's alarm system.

When we ignore it, we are not practicing restraint.

We are silencing a warning.

And in that silence, suffering only grows louder.

In Memory of the Lives Behind the Statistics

Dedicated to everyone lost to addiction — including some of my own patients.

This epidemic did not begin in exam rooms. It began with a narrative.

For years, powerful messaging assured the medical community and the public that certain opioid medications were safe, effective, and carried minimal risk of addiction. Pharmaceutical promotion was confident, persistent, and persuasive. Risks were softened. Benefits were emphasized. A culture formed around rapid symptom relief, and the broader system embraced it.

The consequences were not immediate. They unfolded gradually — prescription exposure increased, surplus medication circulated, and dependence quietly took hold in vulnerable individuals. What followed was not just a prescribing problem; it became a market problem.

As regulations tightened and awareness grew, the supply chain did not disappear — it shifted. Heroin became more accessible. Then fentanyl. Now synthetic opioids dominate the landscape. They are cheap to produce, easy to distribute, and extraordinarily potent. In many communities, illicit opioids are easier to obtain than structured treatment.

This transformation moved the crisis beyond healthcare settings and into neighborhoods, schools, and online spaces.

Our youth were not immune. Counterfeit pills circulate widely. Social media and informal distribution networks lower the barrier to access. Experimentation carries far greater risk today than it did a generation ago. A single exposure can be fatal.

External forces have amplified the problem: economic instability, social fragmentation, untreated trauma, and rising mental health disorders. Addiction rarely exists in isolation. Depression, anxiety, PTSD, and substance use are deeply intertwined. Yet mental health infrastructure has lagged behind the need for decades.

We simply were not prepared.

Treatment resources remain insufficient. In many regions, there are not enough inpatient rehabilitation beds. Intensive outpatient programs are limited. Long-term recovery support is fragmented. Behavioral health access is constrained by workforce shortages and funding gaps. Rural communities feel this most acutely.

When resources are scarce, addiction progresses unchecked.

The impact extends beyond overdose statistics. Families fracture. Children grow up in instability. Workforces shrink. Communities absorb the economic and emotional toll. Individuals struggling with addiction are often marginalized, not because they lack worth, but because untreated illness impairs their ability to function consistently. Society loses potential long before it records a death certificate.

Are we moving in the right direction? There has been progress. Awareness is higher. Naloxone access has expanded. Medication-assisted treatment is more widely accepted. Monitoring systems are stronger.

But overdose deaths remain high, largely driven by illicit synthetic opioids. Mental health systems remain underfunded. Prevention efforts for youth need strengthening. Treatment capacity still does not match demand.

Responsibility is complex, but it is not invisible. Pharmaceutical promotion played a significant role in shaping early perceptions of safety. Illicit drug manufacturing and trafficking networks now fuel ongoing mortality. Policy responses have often been reactive rather than anticipatory. Funding has not consistently matched the scale of the crisis.

This epidemic is not about assigning blame to individual clinicians who practiced within the framework they were given. It is about acknowledging that powerful external forces shaped that framework — and that the downstream consequences have been profound.

To those we have lost — including some of my own patients — your absence is felt. Your stories mattered. You were more than a diagnosis, more than a statistic, more than a chapter in a public health crisis.

If we are serious about honoring those lives, the path forward is clear: sustained investment in mental health, expanded inpatient and outpatient rehabilitation capacity, stronger prevention efforts, and long-term recovery infrastructure. Not temporary attention. Not shifting narratives. Durable commitment.

Addiction is not a moral failure. It is a complex illness amplified by systemic forces. Addressing it requires resources equal to its impact.

That is the responsibility before us now.

The Scalpel and the Clock

Work–life balance. For some, the phrase feels exaggerated, even indulgent. For others, it is a necessary correction to a profession that has long equated exhaustion with virtue. The debate has gained momentum over the past few decades, and it is not a trivial one. At stake are productivity, patient safety, family, identity, and the very soul of medicine.

There was a time when no one spoke of balance. Medicine was not a job to be measured against personal time; it was a calling. The hospital lights were always on. The pager could sound at any hour. Disease did not respect holidays, and neither did the physician. Hard work was assumed. Sacrifice was expected. In many ways, it still is.

To understand the force of this argument, one must understand the making of a doctor. It begins in college, where ambition quietly trades freedom for fluorescent-lit libraries and long nights with textbooks. Medical school is no gentler. The volume of information is staggering, the responsibility sobering. Then comes residency—arguably the most transformative and punishing season. The hours are long, the sleep fragmented, the stakes unbearably high. You learn to deliver life-altering news before you have fully learned to process your own emotions. You function when tired because there is no alternative. You grow, but you also harden.

For generations, this was simply the path. The crucible forged competence and resilience. It shaped physicians who could endure. And the needs were real. Communities lacked doctors. Patients filled emergency rooms. If not you, then who?

Even today, with physician shortages in rural and urban America alike, the argument for relentless commitment carries weight. Medicine demands availability. It is mental work of the highest order—diagnostic reasoning, risk calculation, ethical judgment—all performed often under pressure and uncertainty. It is exhausting, yes, but also deeply rewarding. There is dignity in staying late to stabilize a patient. There is honor in answering one more call. There is meaning in being the steady presence when a family's world is collapsing.

Some physicians never truly separate themselves from this rhythm. I think of a colleague long retired, well into his eighties. Medicine had become part of his blood. Even after stepping down, he continued to help in clinic on a PRN basis. One morning, on his way to work, he suffered a massive stroke and died. He passed away en route to the sacred work he loved. There is something profoundly moving in that image—a life so intertwined with purpose that the boundary between profession and identity disappears.

And yet, there is another image.

An older colleague in his early sixties came into the emergency department not as a physician, but as a patient. Chest pain. His third heart attack. When asked what had happened, he said quietly, "I took care of everyone else and forgot to take care of myself." There was no drama in the statement. Just clarity.

Another colleague spent years in emergency medicine, working long shifts with little sleep. Toward the end of his 24-hour shifts, staff noticed slurring of speech. Concern prompted a workup. He was diagnosed with a rare neurologic condition and ultimately went on disability, forced to leave the profession he had poured himself into. Whether overwork caused his illness is not the point. The point is that exhaustion is not benign. Chronic sleep deprivation is not harmless. The mind that must make life-and-death decisions is still a human mind.

Here lies the counterargument: balance is not laziness. It is stewardship.

We ask physicians to practice safe medicine, to think clearly, to innovate, to lead teams, to comfort families. We cannot ignore that mental fatigue impairs cognition and that chronic stress erodes empathy. A physician who exercises, eats well, sleeps adequately, and has space to breathe is not less committed. He or she may, in fact, be more effective. Mental breaks can sharpen focus. Time with family can restore perspective. A rested mind often works more efficiently than an exhausted one.

Family time is not a trivial luxury. You only see your child at age three once. The bedtime questions, the first recital, the small hand reaching for yours—these moments do not repeat. Many physicians spend their twenties and early thirties postponing life: delaying financial stability, relationships, rest. After college, medical school, and residency—years defined by hours and hours of study and service—it is not unreasonable to hope for a season that allows space for self and family.

It is not wrong for doctors to think about their own well-being. It is not selfish to seek a position with fewer calls, fewer weekends, more sustainable clinic hours. Especially after a decade of relentless training, the desire for balance is understandable—and legitimate. In fact, it may serve patients well. A physician who remains healthy can serve longer. A doctor who avoids burnout may innovate more, lead better, and practice more safely over the span of a career.

Still, the concern remains: if everyone seeks lighter schedules, who carries the load? The workload has not diminished. The shortage persists. The sick still come. Medicine cannot become a profession of convenience. Sacred work requires commitment.

So perhaps the question is not whether sacrifice is good. It is. The question is how much. There must be a limit—not a universal formula, but a thoughtful boundary where devotion does not become self-destruction. Somewhere between the colleague who died on his way to clinic, still serving into his eighties, and the colleague who suffered his third heart attack after forgetting himself entirely, lies a wiser path.

Work–life balance is neither a fad to be dismissed nor a doctrine to be worshiped. It is an ongoing negotiation between calling and capacity. The scalpel and the clock do not have to be enemies. The goal is not less commitment, but sustainable commitment. Not withdrawal from medicine, but longevity within it.

In the end, balance is not about working less. It is about living enough to continue working well. It is about preserving the mind that diagnoses, the hands that heal, and the heart that cares—so that the sacred work of medicine can be done not only intensely, but enduringly.

The Weight of Familiar Faces

There is something no one quite prepares you for in medicine — not in anatomy lab, not in residency, not in leadership courses. It isn't the medicine itself. It's the relationships.

For almost eight years, I practiced in a town of approximately 4,500 people. A traditional practice. The kind that still feels like medicine was meant to feel.

Mornings began before the town fully stirred. Hospital rounds first — quiet hallways, dim lights, patients waking slowly as you adjusted drips, reviewed labs, made decisions that mattered. Then a full day of clinic. One weekend in six. Call every sixth night. ER shifts to keep my edge sharp. Hospitalist work. Coverage for three nursing homes. Driving thirty minutes to round at affiliated facilities. Medical director of two nursing homes. Medical director of the clinic.

It was a full life.

When you come out of residency — after years of relentless pace, sleepless nights, and constant urgency — even a traditional rural practice can feel lighter. You're conditioned to function at a level of exhaustion that feels normal. When that intensity drops, even slightly, you think something is missing. So you take on more — extra shifts, extra responsibilities, extra roles.

Work-life balance is a conversation most of us don't have until much later — after the body whispers, the mind nudges, and the soul quietly asks, Is this sustainable?

After eight years, I transitioned to a full-time ER position in the same geographic area. On paper, it made sense. Focused. Defined shifts. Cleaner boundaries.

But letting go of that clinic was one of the hardest professional decisions I've made.

I had a large number of patients on my panel who called me their PCP and trusted me with their care — not just visits, but their stories. Their fears. Their diagnoses. Their hopes. Over the years, relationships formed not only with patients, but with their spouses, their children — sometimes three generations of the same family. You watched babies grow into teenagers. You cared for aging parents while guiding their adult children through impossible decisions. These were not chart numbers. These were lives woven into your own.

Because our APPs did not round in the hospital, I managed the inpatient care for a few thousand patients across both clinics whenever they were admitted. In the outpatient setting, many saw our APPs and other providers. But if they crossed the threshold into the hospital, they became my responsibility. For a period of time, I was the only MD in our clinic — and the only physician covering all inpatient work for the system. One main clinic. One satellite clinic. A few thousand patients collectively.

The weight of that responsibility was real.

Every admission carried not just clinical complexity, but history. You knew the backstory before opening the chart. You knew which spouse needed extra reassurance. Which family dynamics required careful navigation. Which patient would downplay symptoms. Which one feared the worst.

And they knew you.

They trusted that when they were at their most vulnerable — intubated, septic, frightened, confused — you would be there. A familiar face in an unfamiliar setting.

Walking away from that was not simply leaving a job.

It was stepping away from the role I held within a community — and from a way of practicing medicine — in which I had been entrusted with its most sacred moments: life's beginnings, illness, decline, death.

It has been four years since I left clinic work and transitioned into an ER role, and soon after into an ER/hospitalist position in a different capacity. In this new role, I work only in the hospital. My old clinic is attached to the hospital.

Yet every time I walk back into that clinic, I'm greeted not as a former physician, but as someone returning home.

Hugs. Smiles. Laughter. "When are you coming back?"

"We've kept your spot."

"We still talk about you."

The APPs still call me — case consults, quick questions, reassurance on tough decisions. There isn't a day that goes by that I don't hear from someone there.

And what strikes me most is this: trust doesn't expire.

It endures.

Relationships built on mutual respect and shared struggle do not dissolve when job titles change. They deepen. They become part of your identity.

It feels good to be competent.

It feels good to be effective.

But it feels extraordinary to be trusted.

And even more extraordinary to be loved.

In medicine, we talk endlessly about productivity, RVUs, coverage models, burnout metrics. But rarely do we talk about the invisible architecture that sustains a career — the human connections.

A nurse who knows how you think before you say a word.

A receptionist who protects your schedule because she knows when you need breathing room.

An APP who trusts your judgment without hesitation.

A team that believes you have their back — and knows you believe in them.

That kind of relationship is not built in months. It is forged over years — in shared call nights, in difficult codes, in long clinic days when the waiting room is full and everyone stays just a little longer.

I consider myself fortunate — blessed, really — that in every facility I have worked, I have been met with support and trust. Not because of titles. Not because of authority. But because of consistency, humility, and mutual respect.

Respect is earned in how you speak to people when you're tired.

Trust is built in how you handle mistakes — yours and others'.

Loyalty is formed when people know you will stand with them, not above them.

Medicine can be exhausting. It can be demanding. It can consume more of you than you intended to give.

But when you build profound, meaningful relationships along the way, the work transcends transactions. It becomes shared purpose.

And that is what remains.

Four years later, when I walk into that clinic and see those smiling faces, I'm reminded that our greatest impact is not only in the diagnoses we make or the procedures we perform.

It is in how we made people feel while doing it.

Relationships matter.

They are the quiet legacy of a physician's career.

What Remains After the Applause

What is success in medicine?

Is it the save?

The diagnosis no one else could make?

The septic patient who lives because you saw what others missed?

Is it the hug at discharge? The letter that says, "You changed our lives"?

Or is that just ego dressed up as virtue?

We rarely admit this, but much of what we call success is external. Titles. Leadership roles. Reputation. Being the doctor everyone consults. Being wanted. Being needed. Being indispensable.

But is indispensability the same as success?

Medicine can be identity.

Medicine can be profession.

Medicine can be calling.

Medicine can be job.

Every physician stands somewhere on that continuum. And that place shifts. The resident who swore medicine was a calling may later experience it as a profession. The mid-career physician who treated it as a job may suddenly rediscover it as identity. Life moves us along that spectrum.

Some doctors feel most alive at 2 a.m. in a crashing ICU room. Chaos sharpens them. Responsibility energizes them. They check the EMR on weekends—not because they must, but because they want to. Even on vacation, they wonder about labs, consult notes, outcomes. They cannot disconnect because they do not want to. Medicine is not something they do. It is something they are. Retirement, to them, feels like erasure. They will practice at 80, at 85, because without medicine, they do not quite know who they are.

Others practice with equal competence and compassion—but differently. They give everything during clinic hours. They focus. They care. They show up fully. And then they go home. They close the laptop. They refuse to let medicine colonize their inner life. At 63, they retire without longing. They travel. They read. They garden. They rediscover the parts of themselves that predated the white coat.

Which one is more successful?

The one who cannot live without medicine?

Or the one who can walk away without regret?

We often pretend success is measurable. Income. Rank. Publications. Years practiced. Awards earned. But none of those answer the only question that matters.

When you lie in bed at night, in the dark, without applause, without titles—

are you at peace?

Success in medicine is not linear. It is not diagnostic brilliance alone. It is not perfect work-life balance either. It is alignment—between who you are and how you practice.

Some crave external validation. Others crave internal quiet.

Some need to be needed. Others need to be whole.

The uncomfortable truth?

Both can look identical from the outside.

Two physicians may share the same credentials, the same skill, the same respect among colleagues. One feels deeply fulfilled. The other feels quietly trapped.

So perhaps the real question is not, What is success?

Perhaps it is this:

Is your work an expression of who you are—

or an escape from who you might be without it?

Is success being indispensable?

Or being internally free?

Medicine will take as much of you as you offer. It will reward you with meaning, admiration, gratitude—and sometimes with exhaustion, identity loss, and imbalance. It can become your bloodstream. It can also become your cage.

The criteria for success are not universal. They are intimate. They evolve.

The physician who practices until 85 because medicine is stitched into his DNA may be profoundly successful.

The physician who retires at 63, content and detached, may be equally so.

The difference is not devotion.

The difference is alignment.

So where are you on the continuum?

Medicine as identity?

Medicine as calling?

Medicine as profession?

Medicine as job?

There is no correct answer.

Only this one:

When the day is over, when the noise fades, when the white coat is off—

are you living a life that feels like yours?

From Paper to Pixels

There was a time when medicine rustled.

Charts were thick with paper and history, stacked in long rows of metal shelves. You could feel a patient's story in your hands. Finding a lab meant flipping page by page, deciphering handwriting that only its author truly understood. Hours were spent searching. Errors hid in ink.

Some still speak of those days with longing—quieter clinics, fewer interruptions, no passwords to remember.

But I belong to the generation that barely knew them. In my early training we straddled paper and pixels, and then—almost suddenly—the paper disappeared. The chart became a login. The file room became a server.

Today, a patient's entire story rises in seconds. Labs trend before our eyes. Medications reconcile instantly. Interactions are flagged before harm can occur. What once took hours now takes minutes. Modern medicine, with all its complexity, could not stand without this digital spine.

And yet, the system is imperfect. Not all records speak to one another. Not all platforms are equal. Some hospitals can afford elegance; others must compromise. We have traded illegible handwriting for information overload. Filing cabinets for firewalls.

Working with a computer is not simply typing—it is thinking in layers. Listening to a patient while navigating data, alerts, orders, and documentation. The screen can intrude, but it can also protect. It can fragment attention—or knit together a life-saving detail.

When I chose where to train and practice, the quality of the electronic medical record (EMR) mattered. To my generation, it is not an accessory to medicine. It is its infrastructure.

Paper required space in buildings.

Electronic records require space in our minds.

But the heart of medicine has not changed.

A patient still sits across from us.

A story still needs telling.

A life still rests, quietly, in our hands.

The charts no longer rustle.

They glow.

Smarter Medicine: Why AI Still Needs the Human Brain

Over the past few decades, medicine has gone through a quiet revolution. We moved from paper charts to electronic health records. We adopted templates and smart phrases. We built in automatic safety checks that warn us about medication allergies, dangerous drug interactions, or abnormal lab values. Each step made care safer and more efficient.

Now we are entering the next chapter: artificial intelligence.

Artificial intelligence, or AI, refers to computer systems designed to analyze large amounts of data, recognize patterns, and make predictions or suggestions. It is important to understand what that means—and what it does not mean. AI does not think like a human. It does not have judgment. It does not replace doctors. It is a powerful tool that can process information at speeds and volumes far beyond human capacity, but it does not possess wisdom, experience, or empathy. Those remain uniquely human.

AI is already quietly integrated into many parts of healthcare. An AI system reviewing a chest X-ray may flag a possible pneumothorax and prompt the physician to take a closer look. A CT scanner might detect signs of a brain bleed and immediately alert the emergency team before the radiologist has finalized the report. In these situations, AI does not make the diagnosis. It raises its hand and says, "This may be important." The physician still reviews the images and makes the final decision.

Much like today's electronic records warn us about drug interactions, AI can go further. It can identify subtle patterns suggesting early sepsis, flag lab trends that indicate clinical deterioration, or detect medication dosing risks before harm occurs. These systems act like an extra layer of safety—an assistant quietly monitoring in the background.

AI can also support decision-making at the bedside. It can draw from vast amounts of medical data and research, analyze symptoms, labs, imaging, and history in real time, and offer suggestions about possible diagnoses or treatment options. It can help physicians brainstorm and think through complex cases. But it suggests; it does not decide. The physician remains responsible for interpreting the information and choosing the best path forward.

Some people worry that AI will reduce jobs or replace humans altogether. It is possible that some processes will become leaner and more efficient. But healthcare is fundamentally human. Diagnosis is not just pattern recognition. Treatment is not just an algorithm. Medicine requires judgment, context, ethics, communication, empathy, and accountability. Patients want to be heard. They want someone who understands their fears, values, and personal goals. A machine cannot provide that.

In many ways, AI itself needs a second opinion—from a human. If an algorithm flags a possible stroke on a scan, a physician must confirm it. If AI recommends a treatment pathway, a physician must determine whether it fits the individual patient sitting in front of them. People are more likely to trust a system where a powerful computer analyzes the data and a trained physician reviews and validates the final decision. The combination of machine precision and human judgment is likely the safest model.

The most exciting vision for AI in medicine is not replacement but partnership. We want AI to work alongside physicians in real time, offering suggestions, helping with brainstorming, guiding treatment options, reducing cognitive overload, and improving safety. At the same time, the ultimate decision will always need a human. The human brain remains the final authority.

For patients, this partnership has the potential to mean faster detection of critical findings, fewer errors, more personalized care, and greater efficiency. Ideally, it also frees physicians to spend more time focused on communication and connection rather than paperwork and data management.

We are excited about these advancements. The possibilities are enormous. Medicine is becoming smarter and more responsive. But the future of healthcare is not AI alone. It is AI working with physicians—technology assisting in real time, with human beings ensuring accuracy, safety, and compassion. I may be totally wrong, and this may turn into something very different—something that many people fear—but in my opinion, the most responsible and trusted path forward is one where AI remains a partner, not a replacement. The future is not machine versus human. It is machine and human, working together to provide the best care possible.

Strained, Not Failing: Quiet Victories in American Medicine

Are we doing enough about prevention?

The question lingers in the air, often asked with frustration, sometimes with accusation. It suggests neglect. It implies decay. It assumes that we wait until disease roars before we respond.

But that is not the whole story.

We speak of upstream and downstream, as if medicine were a river. Downstream is loud and visible—ICUs humming, chemotherapy infusing, monitors beeping, specialists intervening when the body has already declared its distress. Upstream is quieter. It is the whispered counsel in a clinic room. The vaccine given without ceremony. The blood pressure checked. The mammogram ordered. The colonoscopy scheduled. The conversation about walking more, smoking less, eating differently, sleeping better.

Downstream makes headlines.

Upstream prevents them.

Yes, our system feels strained. It is caring for a population living longer than any generation before it. Our elderly—wonderfully resilient—are surviving heart attacks, strokes, cancers, infections that once would have ended their stories. Longevity is not failure. It is success with consequences. More years mean more complexity. More chronic disease. More care required.

And so the river grows crowded.

Critics say we wait too long. That we pay dearly when illness is advanced. There is truth there. Prevention requires patience, infrastructure, incentives aligned with the long arc of health. Insurance structures do not always reward investments whose dividends appear decades later. Access is uneven. This is a vast country, layered with differences—economic, cultural, political. Engagement varies. Trust varies. Opportunity varies.

Prevention is not simple. It asks for repetition. It asks for education. It asks for change in habits shaped over a lifetime. It asks for strategy and stamina.

And yet.

Cervical cancer has fallen dramatically, thanks to screening and vaccination. Breast cancer mortality has declined because we detect it earlier and treat it better. Vaccines quietly prevent suffering we rarely see. Colon cancer screening saves lives long before symptoms appear. Blood pressure control prevents strokes that never make the evening news.

This is prevention at work—so effective that its victories are often invisible.

Do not underestimate the doctor who spends five extra minutes discussing weight. The clinician who revisits smoking cessation again and again. The nurse who calls to ensure a patient schedules a mammogram. The primary care visit that catches diabetes early. These are small acts in isolation. Together, they are a force.

Even the obesity epidemic, long a symbol of upstream failure, may be shifting. New tools such as GLP-1 receptor agonists are changing what is possible. We see weight decline. We see metabolic markers improve. We do not yet know the full long-term story, but for now, we see benefit. Combined with lifestyle change, these therapies may alter trajectories once thought fixed.

None of this means we are perfect. We can do better. We must continue pushing earlier, educating more broadly, investing more wisely. We should strengthen community health, reward long-term prevention, and expand access so that geography and income do not determine opportunity.

But let us not confuse strain with collapse. Let us not mistake complexity for failure.

The system is not falling apart. It is carrying a heavier load than ever before. It is caring for older patients, sicker patients, longer-living patients. And still—every day—it vaccinates, screens, counsels, detects early, prevents quietly.

Prevention is not dramatic. It is steady. It is repetitive. It is sometimes thankless.

It is the disease that never develops.

The stroke that never happens.

The cancer found before it spreads.

The habit slowly reshaped.

We can do better. And we will.

But let us also give credit—to the clinicians upstream, speaking into the current, and to the patients who listen and try. In that partnership, prevention lives.

The Unfinished Masterpiece: How Good Is Our Healthcare System?

It's a question that refuses to fade.

The media asks it. Policymakers debate it. Patients wonder about it at kitchen tables. Physicians argue about it in call rooms and conference halls. And depending on who is answering, the verdict ranges from "deeply broken" to "the best in the world."

Both sides are right.

Let's begin with the criticisms, because they are real. The United States spends more per capita on healthcare than almost any nation on earth. Administrative complexity is staggering. Paperwork, prior authorizations, billing layers, compliance mandates, entire ecosystems exist just to move information and money from one column to another. Litigation pressures shape behavior. Defensive medicine inflates costs. Insurance structures and profit models distort incentives. Medication prices frustrate patients and physicians alike. Access remains uneven. Socioeconomic status, geography, and race still influence outcomes. Rural communities struggle. Urban systems overflow.

These are not abstract flaws. They are daily realities.

And yet, that is not the whole story.

To compare the United States healthcare system to that of a small, homogenous Scandinavian country and declare a winner is intellectually convenient, but incomplete. The United States is not a compact social laboratory of five million people with shared culture, narrow income variance, and centralized policy. It is a vast, continental mosaic of 330 million individuals, diverse not only in race and ethnicity, but in language, tradition, wealth, education, ideology, and belief. It contains global financial capitals and rural towns separated by hours of open farmland. It carries staggering innovation and staggering inequality simultaneously.

When you factor in that complexity, the comparison changes.

And then there is the other side of the ledger, the part less frequently emphasized in headline rankings.

Innovation.

There is no country on earth that drives medical innovation like the United States. From mRNA platforms to robotic surgery, from advanced imaging modalities to gene therapies, from AI-driven diagnostics to precision oncology, much of it is born, refined, and scaled here. The most complex surgeries in the world are performed here. The most advanced trauma systems operate here. The breadth of subspecialization available here is unmatched. Diagnostics that would be unavailable or rationed elsewhere are often accessible within hours. Academic centers push boundaries daily. Clinical trials reshape standards of care in real time.

Education? Extraordinary. Research infrastructure? Unparalleled. The density of top-tier academic institutions and teaching hospitals is unmatched globally. The culture of inquiry—of questioning, testing, refining—is deeply embedded in American medicine.

And then there are the physicians.

Walk through a busy emergency department, an academic ICU, a rural critical access hospital, or a cutting-edge oncology center, and you will see clinicians who trained in some of the most rigorous systems in the world. Some came from other nations, drawn by the opportunity to learn, innovate, and practice at the highest level. The global envy is not imaginary. It is measurable—in applications, in fellowships, in collaboration, in investment.

So how do we reconcile these truths?

The American healthcare system is structurally flawed in ways that strain sustainability. Cost inflation, insurance complexity, administrative burden, and inequitable access are not minor blemishes—they are systemic vulnerabilities. They threaten morale. They threaten affordability. They threaten long-term viability.

But those weaknesses do not erase the strengths.

They do not negate the technological leadership.

They do not cancel the research engine.

They do not diminish the clinical excellence.

They do not redefine the skill, dedication, and innovation of American physicians.

The issues that dominate headlines—insurance negotiations, pharmaceutical pricing battles, bureaucratic inefficiencies—are largely structural and financial. They are real, but they are not the same as the quality of the medicine practiced at the bedside. They are not the same as the complexity of the surgeries performed, the sophistication of diagnostic algorithms, the speed at which new therapies move from bench to bedside.

The distinction matters.

Because when we ask, "How good is our healthcare system?" we are often collapsing two separate conversations into one:

- The quality and capability of clinical medicine.

- The structure, financing, and distribution of that medicine.

On the first measure—technology, training, innovation, research depth, procedural complexity—the United States stands at the forefront of modern medicine. On the second—equity, efficiency, affordability, administrative simplicity—we have significant work to do.

Acknowledging the flaws does not weaken the system. It strengthens it. Honest self-assessment is the prerequisite for sustainable excellence. We fix cost structures not because we are failing, but because we are worth preserving. We reform insurance complexity not because our physicians lack skill, but because their skill deserves a system that supports rather than obstructs it.

Perfection is not the starting point. It is the trajectory.

The American healthcare system is not perfect. It is not inexpensive. It is not simple. It is not uniformly equitable. But it is dynamic, innovative, ambitious, and extraordinarily capable. It performs miracles daily—sometimes quietly, sometimes spectacularly.

If we repair the structural inefficiencies, address access disparities, rationalize costs, and align incentives with patient-centered care, we do not become good—we become extraordinary.

The foundation is already there.

The question is not whether American medicine is good.

The question is whether we have the courage to refine a system that is already powerful—so that its excellence becomes accessible, sustainable, and worthy of the innovation it produces.

That is not a story of decline.

It is a story of unfinished potential.

Where I Belong

The question comes often, sometimes casually, sometimes with quiet curiosity: Would you do it again? Would you choose the same specialty?

For me, the answer is a firm and unhesitating yes.

I cannot see myself doing anything else.

Since childhood, science has felt less like a subject and more like a calling. I was the child who visited the doctor often—frequent respiratory infections gave me a familiarity with clinic rooms that most children might dread. But I loved being there. The walls lined with patient education posters, the anatomical illustrations, the crisp paper on the exam table, even the quiet gleam of a syringe resting on a tray— these were not frightening objects to me. They fascinated me. They were symbols. They spoke of knowledge, of healing, of purpose.

I used to tell my mother, with the certainty only a child can have, that I would become a doctor.

While others escaped into novels—and I did too, at times—I found deeper joy in opening a biology textbook. Some might call that boring. I call it the way my mind is wired. Cells, systems, physiology—these were stories to me. Stories written in the language of life itself.

Perhaps part of my love for medicine comes from never imagining myself anywhere else. This is what I know. This is what I have grown into. And that is more than enough.

I love science.

I value human connection.

I find meaning in sitting across from another person and, in some small way, helping lighten their burden. Even if my contribution feels modest, the privilege of being invited into someone's most vulnerable moments brings a satisfaction that is difficult to describe and impossible to replace.

As for specialty, my path was not linear.

Before medical school, I envisioned myself as an ophthalmologist. I had immersed myself in ophthalmic research and developed a deep appreciation for the anatomy and physiology of the eye. The retina—a delicate, curved plate of neurons paired with a lens—remains to me one of the most astonishing creations in biology. A living camera, more sophisticated than anything engineered, translating light into perception. An entire universe contained within a small sphere.

On the first day of medical school, we were asked to write down our intended specialty on a piece of paper. I wrote cardiology. Four years later, when we matched, they returned those same pieces of paper to us. A quiet reminder of who we thought we would become.

Few students truly know at the beginning. Certainty evolves. Exposure refines it. Mentors shape it. Experiences nudge it in unexpected directions.

For me, it was rural rotations that clarified everything.

There, I witnessed medicine in its most complete form—unfiltered and immediate. I saw physicians who were not confined to a narrow lane but practiced broadly, deeply, and courageously. Family medicine in a rural setting is not a job description; it is a commitment. It is continuity. It is first contact, comprehensive care, cradle to grave. It is being present at the front line when there is no one else.

During that time, my passion for rural health crystallized. Family medicine and rural medicine are interwoven—each strengthening the other. The broad scope of practice, the responsibility, the privilege of serving an entire community—these spoke to me more powerfully than any subspecialty ever could.

So yes.

Yes, I would do it again.

Family medicine has not only satisfied me—it has shaped me. It has become part of my identity. This is not employment; it is vocation.

When I take a week or two off, I feel restless. I think about the clinic, the hospital, the patients whose stories are still unfolding. I log in at night or over the weekend, just to check. Not because I must—but because I can't not know. Their lives intersect with mine in meaningful ways, and that connection does not switch off with a schedule.

Medicine is not simply what I do. It is woven into who I am.

If given the choice again, knowing the sacrifices, the weight of responsibility, the long nights, the emotional toll, I would still choose this path. I would still choose family medicine. I would still choose rural health.

In the end, this work allows me to stand at the intersection of science and humanity, to use knowledge in service of people. In small but real ways, it allows me to make a difference.

And there is no greater privilege than that.

About the Author

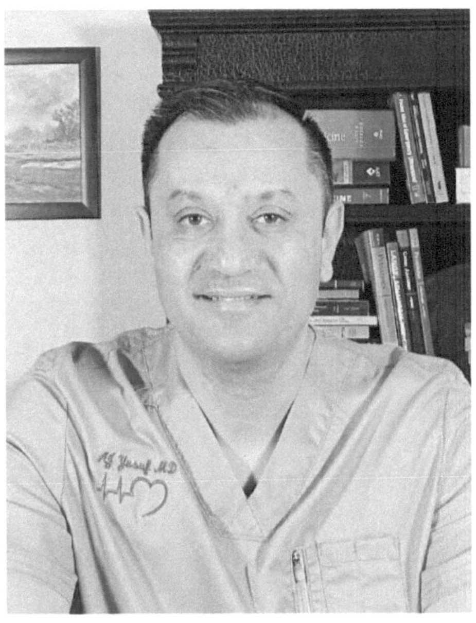

AJ Yusuf, MD, is a family physician and healthcare leader dedicated to reimagining what rural medicine can be. Serving small communities across southwest Minnesota, his work spans clinic, hospital, and emergency care, giving him a front-line perspective on both the challenges and the untapped potential within community healthcare. He believes strong systems are built on trust, accountability, and a shared sense of purpose. Passionate about sustainable innovation and servant leadership, Dr. Yusuf is committed to strengthening rural healthcare so small communities can thrive for generations to come.

To connect with Dr. Yusuf, visit:

LinkedIn: linkedin.com/in/ajyusufmd